OXFORD MEDICAL PUBLICATIONS

An Introduction to Social Psychiatry

An Introduction to Social Psychiatry

A. S. Henderson

National Health and Medical Research Council
Social Psychiatry Research Unit
The Australian National University
Canberra, Australia

OXFORD NEW YORK MELBOURNE
OXFORD UNIVERSITY PRESS
1988

Oxford University Press, Walton Street, Oxford OX2 6DP

Oxford New York Toronto
Delhi Bombay Calcutta Madras Karachi
Petaling Jaya Singapore Hong Kong Tokyo
Nairobi Dar es Salaam Cape Town
Melbourne Auckland
and associated companies in
Berlin Ibadan

Oxford is a trade mark of Oxford University Press

Published in the United States
by Oxford University Press, New York

British Library Cataloguing in Publication Data
Henderson, A.S.
An introduction to social psychiatry.
1. Medicine. Social psychiatry
I. Title
362.2
ISBN 0-19-261637-4
ISBN 0-19-261756-7 Pbk

Library of Congress Cataloging in Publication Data
Henderson, Scott, 1935-
An introduction to social psychiatry / A.S. Henderson.
(Oxford medical publications)
Bibliography:
Includes index.
1. Social psychiatry. I. Title. II. Series.
[DNLM: 1. Community Psychiatry. 2. Mental Disorders—occurrence.
WM 30.6 H497i]
RC455.H46 1988 616.89—dc19 88-12489
ISBN 0-19-261637-4
ISBN 0-19-261756-7 (pbk.)

Set by The Alden Press, Oxford
Printed in Great Britain by
Biddles Ltd, Guildford and King's Lynn

Preface

To all who want to learn about the causes and management of mental disorders, social psychiatry now offers a rich store-house of information. Its viewpoint is also an essential complement to knowledge about the biological basis of mental disorders; and it necessarily will always remain so. In this book, I have given an overview of the field encompassed by social psychiatry, in the hope that it will serve as a useful starting point for readers. If I am fortunate, it may even infect some readers with the enthusiasm I caught from my own teachers in Edinburgh, particularly Morris Carstairs and Norman Kreitman, and from my father for a concern with public health. Since these years, social psychiatry has proved to be an engaging subject.

I am fully aware that the coverage in this book is far from complete. Nothing has been included, for example, on drug abuse or mental retardation; and the coverage of both forensic and transcultural psychiatry is very limited. These are topics which have now been adequately covered in other volumes, and in which I have had no clinical or research experience.

I much appreciate the help of many friends and colleagues while preparing this book. The greatest contribution has been by Dr Paul Bebbington, who critically read the manuscript over several months, and alerted me to important omissions and errors. No doubt many of these remain, but he appreciably reduced them, and was unsparing in his help. Professor P. A. P. Moran, FRS and Dr Anthony Jorm also commented constructively on the text. In specific areas, I have been grateful to Professor Gavin Andrews, Dr James C. Anthony, Dr John Birtchnell, Professor Tony Broe, the late Mr Paul Duncan-Jones, Prof. David Guldberg, Dr David Grayson, Professor Dr Dr H. Häfner, Professor Assen Jablensky, Professor D.W.K. Kay, Professor Leslie Kiloh, Dr Julian Leff, Professor Gordon Parker, Professor Issy Pilowsky, Dr Michael Power, Dr Stephen Rosenman, Professor Michael Rutter, Dr Norman Sartorius, Professor Michele Tansella, Dr Christine Vaughn, Dr Paul Williams, Professor John Wing, and Dr Lorna Wing. Ms Karen Maxwell and Mrs Penny Evans, our Unit secretaries in Canberra, prepared the text and index on diskettes, doing so with accuracy, persistence, and good humour. I much appreciate their contribution. To Dr Sarah Hnatiuk and Mrs Ruth Scott, I am particularly grateful for their work with the secretaries on the text, references and index. Throughout, I have been supported by the National Health and Medical Research Council at The Australian National University. While on leave in the United Kingdom in 1987, I was given every possible assistance and support by the MRC Social Psychiatry Unit at the Institute of Psychiatry, Maudsley Hospital, and by the Medical Research Council. The greatest stimulus and encouragement, though, came from my wife Priscilla, and from Mhairi, Susan, Calum, Catriona, and Angus.

Canberra A.S.H.
January 1988

Contents

1

Introduction

Social psychiatry is concerned with the relationship between disorders of the mind and the human environment. It studies the forces which act at the interface between individuals and those around them; and which may contribute to the onset, or influence the course of mental disorders. The social environment extends from immediate others, as in the family, to the wider society. The word social originates from the Latin *socius*, meaning a companion. This in turn may derive from the Vedic *sakka*, with the same meaning (Partridge 1966). For the purposes of psychiatry, the term 'social' can be thought of as having two components. The first refers to the interaction between a person and all those who populate his or her life, both in the past and at present. This personal network or what Cooley (1909) called the primary group, extends from close, intimate relationships to brief and superficial encounters in daily life. It is the person's social world. It is World 2 in Karl Popper's scheme, in contrast to the physical world (World 1) and the world of the mind (World 3) (Popper 1972). But there is a second level of the social environment, which is considered likely to be highly relevant for mental disorders and mental well-being. It is much more abstract and includes constructs such as social cohesion, shared values, economic conditions, threat by an enemy, and the expectation of survival. These are macrosocial phenomena, sometimes difficult to define with precision or to measure, but nevertheless attributes of a society which certainly influence behaviour in daily life and which may promote or inhibit some types of mental disorder. These phenomena are what the early social scientist, Durkheim (1897), examined when developing concepts such as 'anomie' or normlessness. They continue to be considered when comparisons of morbidity are made between populations or ethnic groups.

Here we shall examine what is known about social influences on mental health, and how this body of knowledge is coming to form a coherent pattern, based on contributions which have been accumulating throughout this century. Social psychiatry has developed into a robust arm of medical research and practice for at least two reasons.

First, mental disorders have for long been considered to be induced or exacerbated by happenings in the social environment. In primitive societies, the attribution has commonly been to the malignant influence of spirits. This has now given way to a belief in the pathogenic effect of factors in the actual social environment. Forces outside the individual are thought likely to have a powerful effect in causing mental disorders; and only in the last few decades has it become possible to examine this general hypothesis systematically. The pressure to do so has been considerable, because the paradigm is congruent with that widely held in industrialized societies—that the origin of most human ills lies in social conditions—a paradigm we shall look at critically. Secondly, more than in any other branch of medicine, it is psychiatry which has made impressive progress in investigating the fabric of the social environment, and in harnessing it for treatment. A similar attention to social phenomena has not been seen elsewhere in the practice of medicine. The consequence is that social psychiatry has been able to make some major contributions to both methods and knowledge in the health sciences, as in its exploration of the effects of adversity on health, of help-seeking and pathways to care, of social factors in the outcome of disorders and in rehabilitation from chronic illness.

Social psychiatry is of course only one component of a wider body of knowledge about mental disorders. It complements three other fields: psychopathology, which seeks to understand how behaviour, cognition and emotional processes are affected in mental illness; biological psychiatry with its focus on the neurosciences and genetics; and clinical psychiatry, which over the last hundred years has accumulated a rich stock of information about the actual phenomenology of mental disorders, their onset, course, and treatment. As one of these four sectors, social psychiatry has a vital integrative role. Whatever the advances we can anticipate in the biological field, the social environment will always remain indispensable, both for diagnosis and for treatment.

Psychiatry as a whole has really only one principal aim: to reduce suffering from mental disorders. All of the above fields are to be seen as united in this common objective. On occasion, the one field may generate ideas or findings which another can profitably develop. In this way, social psychiatry stands as a reminder that indeed no man is an island, that molecular events in brain cells have repercussions on the person's social environment; and that, reciprocally, such molecular events may at times be influenced by happenings in the environment.

The working agenda in social psychiatry consists of *those experiences taking place between people which may influence their mental health.* This sentence specifies the three main sets of variable which have to be considered, whether in research or in the clinical practice of social psychiatry: the social experiences and other social variables; the characteristics of the persons; and the nature of the psychiatric morbidity. In Chapter 2, 'The tools of social psychiatry', an account is given of the methods used to obtain some of this information. We shall argue that social psychiatry has done well both in investigating social experiences and in measuring morbidity; but it has neglected the characteristics of the person, to its detriment.

The simplest approach has been the *naturalistic observation* of patients, describing a clinical state in its social context, and how it is believed to have come about. Individual case studies are a special example of this method. Freud used it exclusively, concluding that the social or interpersonal context was insufficient to explain the onset of disorders, and that forces at work within the individual's mind had to be invoked to provide a satisfactory explanation. It is well-known that he took a major step in deciding that his patients' self-reported sexual experiences were not pathogenic life-events in their own right, but were distortions of their immediate social worlds. In doing so, he moved from a search for an exclusively environmental aetiology to propose largely intrapsychic explanations. Naturalistic observation of the *actual* social context of mental disorders remains a legitimate starting point if we want to try to understand causal processes.

The next approach in social psychiatry has been to assemble data on a series of patients, and to search for a general pattern in this aggregation. The most developed form of this approach is the *case register*, which usually refers to treated morbidity in a defined catchment area. When a comparison is made between patients and those not afflicted with a particular disorder, a *case-control study* is being conducted. Lastly is the epidemiological *field survey*, where the investigator tries to study mental disorders as they exist in the general population, not just in those who reach treatment. Both the case-control study and the field survey require measurement of illness and of possibly relevant experiences. Chapter 2 examines how mental disorders are measured, an area in which progress has been so considerable in recent years; and how aetiological variables, such as stressors or social support, can be quantitatively assessed.

To assemble the knowledge flowing from such research, and for its exposition in this book, we have found it helpful to construct a heuristic device. This is presented in Chapter 3 as '*A matrix for organizing epidemiological knowledge*'. Experience in teaching trainees in public health, psychiatry, and clinical psychology indicates that this matrix serves a useful purpose. It helps to put order into a sizeable field; it prompts one's memory about cells or associations which might otherwise have been ignored, and it generates important questions which our minds might not spontaneously identify. The matrix is set out in Tables 3.1 and 3.2 on pp. 31 and 34.

This sets an agenda, which is begun in Chapter 3, on 'Epidemiological knowledge about mental disorders'. The chapter systematically goes through the information which is available on the distribution of mental disorders by the major sociodemographic variables, but also on their occurence in different world regions and their changing frequency over time. Chapter 4 continues the agenda in the matrix, considering those experiences in life which may be related to psychiatric morbidity. Here, an account is given of areas in social psychiatry which have been accorded much attention, such as life-event research and the current interest in social support. The complementary side of social psychiatry is the social consequences of mental illness. This is discussed in some detail in Chapter 5.

Because of the importance of general practice and primary care in the provision of mental health services, considerable attention has been given to this area in Chapter 6. Much has been learned in recent years about what happens when a person with psychological symptoms seeks help from a general practitioner, how well the symptoms are recognized, and what usually follows in terms of treatment. This is reviewed and the prospects for further progress are examined.

Chapter 7 considers the application of knowledge from social psychiatry to patient care, including prevention. There is already available a large amount of information which, if fully used, could lead to the prevention of much disability. This leads directly in Chapter 8 to the principles used in evaluating services, where a great deal can be done to make better use of available resources.

Finally, we have tried in Chapter 9 to look at where social psychiatry now stands and where the growing points are likely to lie.

At a time when rapid progress is being made in biological psychiatry, an awareness of what is known in the social domain is now needed for a balanced understanding of mental disorders. This book provides an outline of that territory; and one hopes it will encourage readers to become interested in issues which have such importance for public health.

2

The tools of social psychiatry: its methods and instruments

Methods: studies based on clinical impressions; case studies; the analysis of records; the epidemiological paradigm; case-control studies; population surveys; cross-sectional and cohort designs; instruments for measuring morbidity; the concept of a case; the range of independent (possibly causal) variables.

Social psychiatry uses a range of well-established strategies to obtain knowledge about mental illness and the social environment. These are its *methods* for exploring this relationship. The *instruments* are the tools used to determine, more or less systematically, that a particular psychiatric disorder is present; or that a particular attribute of the social environment is present now, or was so in the past. We shall start this chapter by looking at the range of methods, then go on to consider the instruments for measuring morbidity and the crucial concept of a 'case'. This sets the scene for us then to ask how the body of knowledge in social psychiatry can be organized in our minds; what is the territory to be explored; and what research questions can be posed which will benefit patient care and the public health.

STUDIES BASED ON CLINICAL IMPRESSIONS

The starting point for advancing knowledge in social psychiatry, as elsewhere in medicine, has often been in the mind of an alert clinician engaged in the care of patients. Gruenberg calls this process 'from practice to theory'; and his own recognition of the social breakdown syndrome in mentally ill persons is such an example (Gruenberg 1974). What he observed in the course of routine clinical work in a mental hospital led him to construct a theory about the induction of disability in patients' social performance (see p. 107). In such naturalistic observations, the investigator derives an idea about aetiology from within an assembly of facts and impressions. Some of this process is intuitive, but he is often much influenced by a contemporary paradigm. The idea has then to be fashioned into a testable hypothesis. That hypothesis usually involves emphasis being placed on a particular part of all the phenomena being observed, with an explanation which is consonant with a currently popular paradigm. Examples are Bowlby's observations on children in residential nurseries (Bowlby 1977*a*, *b*), the notion of clustering of adversity and illness (Hinkle and Wolff 1975*a*), Lidz's proposals about the families of schizophrenics (Lidz *et al.* 1958; Lidz 1964) and the buffering effect of social ties proposed by Cassel (1976). Bowlby described the emotional and behavioural changes in young children when they are separated from their mothers, proposing that the separation leads not only to distress at the time, but also to a greatly increased vulnerability to depression in adult life (see Chapter 4). Hinkle and Wolff found that people have a much increased probability of falling ill immediately after experiencing adverse life-events. Lidz proposed, erroneously as it turned out, that the families of schizophrenics communicated in a manner which caused the onset of schizophrenic symptoms in their afflicted member. Cassel saw a component in the wider social environment which was supportive, and which he proposed acted as a cushion or buffer against adversity, thereby protecting against some forms of physical morbidity. In each of these, external events or experiences have been thought to influence the mental health of the individual. Attributes of the host were thought *not* to be a prominent issue. These examples illustrate how confrontation with clinical phenomena can generate a new idea in an alert observer, an idea which then has to be more formally tested on fresh evidence.

CASE STUDIES

Instead of waiting for an idea to emerge after lengthy exposure to clinical work, another approach is deliberately to make a detailed study of only a few individuals, noting in detail the antecedents and the current social and cultural context. Such an idiographic approach, conducted by a trained observer interacting intensively with informants, can be useful for gaining insights into the processes at work (idiographic: 'relating to the study of individual cases'—*Dictionary of behavioral science*, edited by Wolman 1973). It has the capacity to produce richly detailed information on the personal and social worlds of the persons observed. This can then be used to generate hypotheses for testing under conditions less open to bias, particularly the distorting effects of case selection. Critics of the case study approach point out that the information obtained, however plausible and appealing, is necessarily based on only a few cases; and that there must be many others who show the same social phenomena but no mental disorder; or who have the disorder though they have not been exposed to the same social phenomena. These issues are better tackled by epidemiological methods, which are essentially nomothetic, meaning 'referring to methods and procedures used to formulate general laws or statements' (Wolman 1973). Case studies are nevertheless a legitimate starting point, provided they lead to the setting up of refutable hypotheses.

THE ANALYSIS OF RECORDS

Information on social factors and mental disorders can sometimes be obtained from data collections which already exist. These will necessarily refer only to persons who have reached treatment. If the selection effect is considered not too damaging, treated rates can then be studied in relation to variables which reflect some social factor. An example is the celebrated work of Goldhamer and Marshall (1953) in their book *Psychosis and civilization*, which examined admission rates for psychosis to Massachusetts mental hospitals for one hundred years from 1840. They were investigating the truth of the belief that mental illnesses had increased in frequency, due to the pressures of modernization. Goldhamer and Marshall did find a marked increase in admission rates, but when they went on to examine these by age-group, the picture changed: it was only in persons aged over 50 years that the increase was striking. This increase, they thought, was largely attributable to a change in social habits, whereby families no longer invariably cared for their elderly with dementias. In his volume on *The sociology of mental disorders*, Eaton (1980) has since pointed out that Goldhamer and Marshall may have attended selectively to the data available, and have not produced satisfactory evidence that rates have remained much the same. He quotes more recent data on service utilization by Morton Kramer which shows a massive increase in treated episodes of psychiatric disorders between 1946 and 1973 in the United States (from 629 to 2508 episodes per 100 000 population) (Kramer 1983). These studies are an example of mental health records' being put to sound scientific use, even though the data did not allow testing of the central hypothesis about increasing rates of mental disorder in the general population.

There have been other studies which relate routinely collected rates to macrosocial factors or changing social conditions. Hare (1983) has made a sound case for the hypothesis that schizophrenia has become more common in the last hundred and fifty years, basing his evidence on hospital admission rates (see p. 62 *et seq.*). Death rates from cirrhosis of the liver have been used as an index of alcohol abuse. An association has been found between suicide rates and the economic depression of the 1930s (WHO 1982*a*). Using official records of death by suicide, Sainsbury (1955) conducted a classic study of the distribution of suicide rates in London boroughs, showing that these were linked to features in the social ecology of each borough. For over a quarter of a century, Krupinski and his colleagues have used a case register in Victoria, Australia, to study patterns of psychiatric morbidity in that State. This has included a comparison of rates in migrants with the rest of the community (Krupinski 1967, 1984).

In all of these studies, what is observed may not be representative of the true pattern in the whole population. This applies both to naturalistic and case studies because of the particular persons who happen to be observed and the validity of their reports, given to a single, highly motivated observer. It is the same criticism as made by Freeman (1983) in his study of Margaret Mead's social anthropological work in Samoa. Investigators tend to find what they expect to find. But similar limitations also apply to data obtained from hospital services, because important groups will not have reached that level of care. Such work need not be spurned, though, provided one remains alert to the ways in which the information derived may be incomplete. The degree of incompleteness may indeed be trivial. Over-concern with such imperfections in the data may blind the investigator to the real value of what does lie in his material.

Those who recognize the place of idiographic studies find themselves inevitably at odds with epidemiologists, whose approach is essentially nomothetic. The latter can indeed achieve representative samples and be aware of the sources of biased information; but they cannot come to grips with the biographic and contextual factors in each member of a sample of several hundred persons. So each approach should be seen to complement the other. The tension between the two approaches and the merits of each have been well appreciated by G. W. Brown and his colleagues (see pp. 85 and 100), who have attempted to import to epidemiological research some of the strengths of the idiographic method. They achieve this, though, by being prepared to conduct interviews lasting five hours or more, sometimes repeated over the course of a year.

THE EPIDEMIOLOGICAL PARADIGM

As soon as the investigator starts to be interested in the distribution of a disorder in the general population, in contrast to its features only in those who have reached services, a transition in scientific method has been made: this is now epidemiology. It uses an appealingly clear-minded style of thinking about causal processes in the onset and outcome of diseases. The word literally means 'around' (*epi*) 'the people' (*demos*). Epidemiology is concerned with how diseases are distributed in populations; and what factors influence this distribution (Lilienfeld 1957). A succinct definition by Greenwood (1935) is that epidemiology examines 'the mass aspects of disease'. For readers unfamiliar with the language of epidemiology, a useful reference is *A dictionary of epidemiology* (Last 1983), in which definitions and brief descriptions will be found for many of the terms used in this book.

The key to the epidemiological way of thinking—and indeed its greatest strength—is captured in the single question, 'What is the true numerator and the true denominator out of which these observations are derived?' This will yield a rate: so many persons (cases) per hundred or per thousand. The rates most commonly used are of incidence and of prevalence. The *incidence* (*syn.* inception) rate is the number of new cases appearing in a population, usually in one year. It may have to be specified whether this refers to persons falling ill for the first time, or if the count includes relapses. The *prevalence* rate is the number of persons suffering from a given disorder in a specified time, again usually a year. For chronic disorders, such as dementia or schizophrenia, the incidence (if it can be estimated) will be low, but the prevalence much higher. That is because prevalence = incidence × duration of the illness. Figure 2.1 sets out diagrammatically the difference between incidence and prevalence, and why it is necessary to distinguish between persons and episodes.

The question about the true numerator should always be asked regarding the cases being studied: if the clinical features are not representative of all the cases which have occurred in that population, erroneous conclusions may be drawn. The same question may

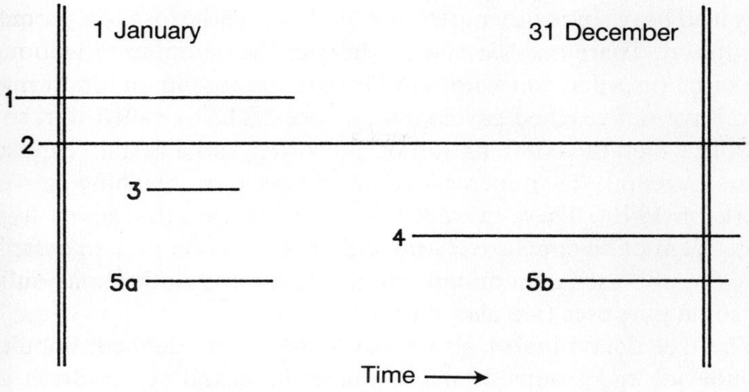

Fig. 2.1 The difference between incidence and prevalence.

1. Case going into remission;
2. Chronic case;
3. Incident case (brief episode);
4. Incident case (longer episode);
5. Relapsing case (two inceptions in one year).

One-year incidence: 4 cases or episodes (Nos 3, 4, 5a, and 5b)
3 persons (Nos 3, 4, and 5).

One-year prevalence: 6 cases or episodes (1, 2, 3, 4, 5a, and 5b)
5 persons.

equally well be asked of the independent variables, such as a particular social experience. For example, to determine if mental health tends to be impaired in the year following bereavement, it is not satisfactory to conduct the study only on those psychiatric patients who have had a recent bereavement. The same experience will have befallen many others who do not become psychiatric, let alone general practice patients. An illustration of the hazards of aetiological research on treated cases is in the extensive literature on maternal separation or loss in childhood and depressive illness in adult life. It is not sufficient to look for this association only in persons who have reached psychiatric services. Childhood loss, or other variables linked to that experience, may themselves be associated with seeking help or being in contact with psychiatric services. That is, persons with a particular disorder may be more likely to have reached psychiatric care if, in addition to the disorder, they also have some other attribute, in this case the loss of a parent in childhood. There may be many others in the community who have the same disorder, but who had no parental loss in childhood, and who have not reached psychiatric services. This is called Berkson's bias, in which the combination of a disorder and a certain exposure (here parental loss) increases the chances of reaching services (Berkson 1946). These examples forcibly indicate that many hypotheses cannot be conclusively upheld or rejected on patient samples: only the unbiased denominator of a general population may suffice for some purposes (see also Eaton 1975).

The true denominator also needs to be clearly defined. Should it include all age-groups in the population, including children; and should it include special groups, such as vagrants, or those in institutional care, in schools, prisons, or the armed services? These may be omitted from the denominator, but may contain many persons who suffer from the disorder, or who have the independent variables in question. An estimate of the denominator can usually be obtained from local census data. But in some communities, particularly in developing countries, this may not be available. It is then necessary to do one's own census. A useful way of remembering the foregoing is to think of a 2×2 table, made up of numerator/denominator and the dependent/independent variables.

What is the relationship between epidemiology and social psychiatry? The two have had a close association because the methods of epidemiology have proved so relevant to the search for aetiological clues in the social environment. Epidemiology has developed methods for screening populations for psychiatric or medical disorders, and methods for identifying groups at increased risk. Also, epidemiology offers methods for evaluating services, how they are being used, and how resources can best be deployed. Lastly, in conducting its business, epidemiology is able to embrace all possible factors, whether these be social, personal or biological. Social psychiatry, by contrast, focuses mainly on environmental and experiential factors.

At first inspection, there may seem to be a bewildering range of designs in epidemiology, but confusion can be avoided by imaging a time-stream of events befalling a population. At the start of the observations, it can be assumed to be healthy, or those already suffering from the disorder in question can be excluded. But members of the population will already differ in their biological and psychosocial attributes. As time passes, and as the population is exposed to various experiences or agents, some will develop certain diseases, including the one of interest. The epidemiologist wants information about this process of pathogenesis, and if he is investigating services, he wants to know what subsequently happens to those afflicted.

For research on disease aetiology, the outcome of disorders, or use of services, there are basically two approaches. One can see this metaphorically as the use of a camera. If only one picture is taken, it is a snapshot of the here-and-now, and is either a case-control study or a cross-sectional population survey. The researchers try to reconstruct the past experiences of those in the picture, to account for whether they are now well or ill. But if subsequent pictures are taken, the design becomes a prospective longitudinal or cohort study, in which the particular focus is on those who develop symptoms during the period of observation, having been well when baseline measures on them were made. Clearly, a prospective design is very expensive and labour-intensive; and the results come only after a substantial period has elapsed. It should be noted, too, that prospective longitudinal studies are only a series of snapshots, not a cine-film. There is no equivalent for the latter in psychiatric epidemiology: what causal processes have taken place in the intervals between the serial snapshots have still to be inferred. Such an issue comes to be highly relevant, for example, in research on depression, life-events and social support.

If a description of a series of patients is to mean much, it should usually be contrasted with at least one other group. Gruenberg's aphorism is that a study without a control group is like a compass without a needle: it will lead you anywhere you point it. Descriptions of clinical series fortunately often do have a comparison group, and therefore have some of the characteristics of a more formal case-control study. But there are times when it can be useful to conduct only a *descriptive study* initially, reporting the clinical, social or other characteristics of a comprehensive sample of patients. Their clinical features should always be well-specified, so that others can be clear about the type of disorder which was investigated. There may be no comparison group in such a study, because the experiential characteristics of the patients may be so obviously distinct. An example can be found in the literature on survivors of the Nazi holocaust or other extreme experiences.

CASE-CONTROL STUDIES

The most economical and direct way to investigate social aetiologies is the case-control method. It is not necessary to screen a total population to identify the cases in it, which is a very expensive procedure. Instead, one may be prepared to assume that cases reaching the services, and therefore at least notionally available to the investigator, will be representative of all those occurring in a population; or that selection effects acting on those chosen will apply equally to the controls. The purpose of the case-control study is to find what experiences or exposures have contributed to the development of a disease. The design for this is essentially very straightforward. A series of cases is compared with a control group of similar size who resemble the cases except that they have not, at least yet, developed the disorder. If certain experiences or exposures have taken place more often in the cases, these may have contributed to its onset. Such a comparison is disarmingly simple, because to undertake a good case-control study is exceedingly demanding: it is necessary all the time to anticipate how biases might unwittingly enter in the collection of the cases, of the control individuals, and of the information obtained about both groups. Some very readable descriptions of these issues are now available (Lilienfeld and Lilienfeld 1980; Ibrahim and Spitzer 1979; Schlesselman 1982; Anthony, (1988). The essential requirements are listed below, but readers will find that many other important issues, both in design and analysis, are brought out in these texts. The following five points need particularly close attention.

1. The cases should be representative of all *incident* cases occurring in the population during the study period. If they are not truly representative of all the cases occurring, it could be that those taken into the study have some special characteristics which have increased the chances not of their developing the disorder, but of entering the study. If prevalent cases are taken instead of fresh or incident ones, some attributes may be found in the cases which really have more to do with *surviving* after developing the disorder than with its primary aetiology. This is sometimes called Neyman's bias. It may therefore be important in the data collection to estimate the time which had elapsed between the onset of the disorder and entry into the study,

then to see if an association exists between this lapse time and any of the putative risk factors.

2. The cases should really have the disorder being investigated, and not something else or something similar. Where certainty about diagnosis during life can be difficult, as for example in senile dementia of Alzheimer type, this requirement can be hard to meet. Calculations can be made, though, about the effect of misclassification on the estimate of relative risk (see below), so that this uncertainty about diagnosis can be allowed for, by increasing the sample size.

3. The controls should either be matched one-for-one with the cases; or be similar overall in attributes such as age, sex, and sometimes other sociodemographic factors. But over-matching can cheat the investigator of an opportunity to detect a risk factor: a difference between cases and controls which really exists can be removed by such matching. Non-matched designs have become more attractive since the introduction of logistic regression methods. These can make the recruitment of controls a little easier through placing fewer constraints on the attributes they have to fulfil. It can be tedious and sometimes very difficult to find controls who are well-matched in age, sex, social class, and other attributes. There are now statistical ways to avoid this, and at the same time to avoid unwanted variation for the analysis.

4. It is often likely that more information will be produced about the cases than about the controls. This may be generated by the patients through the important process of 'effort after meaning' to account for their illness (Bartlett 1932; Brown and Harris 1978), or by their relatives in giving a history, for essentially the same reason. Both parties may feel obliged to account for the illness in terms of experiences. For example, there are reports that elderly persons with Alzheimer's disease have had a head injury, often in much earlier adult life, more often than controls. But this could be due to their relatives' recalling such events more eagerly than the controls' relatives, to account for the dementia. Information bias may also be due to more assiduous interviewing by the investigators, who may find themselves extracting more information from those with the condition in which the interest lies. It is rarely possible to 'blind' the interviewers on whether the respondent is a case or a control. This can be a major source of biased information.

5. The numbers of cases required to show an effect from some

exposure should ideally be calculated beforehand. This can be determined by establishing the minimum size of the effect to be demonstrated; and the frequency with which *controls* have been exposed to the factor in question. Clearly, the more common the exposure in the general population, the more cases will be required for a causal effect to be suggested. Tables for making such estimates have been provided (e.g. Schlesselman 1982).

One should try to bear constantly in mind that the collection of data in a case-control study is towards one specific purpose: to obtain information on the previous history and exposure of both cases and of controls, so that there is some likelihood of finding what noxious experience has happened more often to the cases. That experience can then reasonably be proposed as a likely contributor to the onset of the disease.

The assessment of risk The strength of this contribution is commonly expressed by one of three statistics: the relative risk, the odds ratio and the attributable risk. Particularly clear explanations of these terms can be found in MacMahon and Pugh (1970, p. 232 *et seq.*) and Schlesselman (1982, pp. 32–4; 40–2). To calculate these three statistics, one starts with the information in a 2×2 table, for which Table 2.1 is the prototype. This shows the frequency (a) with which cases develop over a given time (the incidence) in persons exposed to a certain risk factor; and the incidence (c) in those not exposed. This is compared to the number of non-afflicted persons who were exposed (b), and the number who were not exposed (d). The *relative risk*, R, is the ratio of the incidence rate in those exposed to those not exposed in the total population. It is nearly always estimated on only a sample of that population; and that sample often

Table 2.1 A 2×2 table in a case-control study (the letters refer to numbers of persons)

	Cases	Not cases
Exposed	a	b
Not exposed	c	d

consists only of those who have reached a teaching hospital. The biases which this may introduce could lead to mistaken conclusions, and deserve to be thought through in some detail in every study. The relative risk is calculated from Table 2.1 as follows:

$$\frac{a}{a+b} \div \frac{c}{c+d}$$

By simple algebra, this can be reduced to:

$$\frac{a(c+d)}{c(a+b)}$$

Now something very simple but helpful can be done. Where a disorder is fairly uncommon in the population, (a) will be very small in comparison with (b); and (c) small in comparison with (d). By assuming a negligible contribution by (a) in the term $(a+b)$, or (c) in the term $(c+d)$, the relative risk will be nearly equal to:

$$\frac{ad}{bc}$$

This is the *odds ratio* and can be determined both from a case-control and a cohort study (Schlesselman 1982). Indeed, a case-control study can usually estimate only the odds ratio. It is not uncommon for authors mistakenly to use prevalence rates for this calculation in place of incidence. This can be misleading if the risk factor is somehow associated with survival after contracting the disorder.

These two statistics, relative risk and odds ratio, may not give all the information one wishes. For example, with some fairly unusual disorder, a relative risk or odds ratio may be found which is numerically the same as for a much more common one. The relative risks may both be, say, 5, but the public health implications very different. For example, suppose that becoming unemployed confers a relative risk of 4.5 for developing a major depression; and also a relative risk of 4.5 for developing an obsessive-compulsive neurosis. Clearly, the former state has a much greater implication for public health, because major depression is more common. The third statistic, *attributable risk*, is defined as the difference between the incidence rates in those exposed and not exposed. It is an expression of how much the incidence would be reduced if that risk factor were removed from the population. This requires one to have extra information *from outside the case-control study*, to know what the base rate for the disorder is in the general population. This cannot be adequately estimated from the sample of cases and non-cases in a case-control study. But it can be calculated from incidence data in a population survey. An easily read account of this is given by Lilienfeld and Lilienfeld (1980, p. 217). The relative risk is a more revealing statistic if one is mainly interested in the strength of an association. Attributable risk, on the other hand, is more relevant for prevention through public health action.

Application of the case-control method to social psychiatry These expressions of association have been under-used in social psychiatry, probably because many clinical researchers have not been familiar with case-control methods until quite recently. In aetiological work, estimates of relative and attributable risk are strongly to be recommended as complementary to estimates of explained variance. (Variance is a measure of the amount of variation in a set of scores. To 'explain' variance is to be able to account for this variation in terms of all the other, independent variables measured. See, for example, Armitage and Berry 1987.) As we shall see (Chapter 4), life events have been said to contribute only about 10 per cent to the variance in psychiatric morbidity. This could mislead some into thinking their effect was fairly trivial, but Paykel (1978) showed that life-events nevertheless confer a relative risk of between 2 and 7 for psychiatric disorders, which is a substantial effect. The two statistics are in fact congruent.

It is certain that the case-control method should be used more often for aetiological research in social psychiatry. Most psychiatric disorders have a relatively low incidence in the general population, so that using the survey approach requires large numbers to be screened to identify an unbiased sample of incident cases. This is labour-intensive and costly. If only incident cases are to be used, the population sample has to be very large indeed. By contrast, a case-control study makes efficient use of patients already identified, and can allow one to look for interaction effects. Schlesselman (1982, p. 18) provides a convenient list of the strengths and disadvantages compared to what cohort studies offer.

POPULATION SURVEYS

If one wants to learn how indeed diseases are distributed in a population and what factors influence that distribution, sometimes only a survey can reveal this, because for some disorders only a survey can give an unselected sample of cases. As we have already stressed, data from services may tell an incomplete story and even be misleading. For example, case registers may reveal much about the use of services and the outcome in those treated by them, but there may be other cases in the true numerator (the number of cases actually present in the population); and these will not have been included in the case register. Some of those may have sought professional help, as from general practitioners, and not be included in the case register. For disorders such as neurosis, we know that as few as 1 in 20 cases known to general practitioners are referred for consultation to psychiatric services (Shepherd *et al.* 1981). An issue of great interest is the real clinical significance of those 'cases' identified in a survey who have not reached services, particularly where the latter are readily available. Not enough is known about them, although Tennant *et al.* (1981) found in the second Camberwell Survey that many had only transient symptoms.

Although the population survey is the methodological ideal, there are often occasions when it is not practicable. This can be because a survey would prove prohibitively expensive, such as one setting out to identify all cases of a fairly rare condition, for example obsessive-compulsive neurosis. Secondly, there are occasions when it is reasonable to assume that cases reaching treatment are likely to be nearly all those in the community, as it would be for, say, acute mania. Here case registers would be an efficient and methodologically accepted alternative to population surveys.

Note that the choice between a case-control study and a population survey is not mutually exclusive: provided the yield of cases is large enough, a case-control study can be *nested* inside a survey, the controls being derived from those who are found to be healthy.

A population survey should have at least four components: a clear aim, or even a hypothesis; a population with defined geographic and demographic boundaries; a standardized method for case-finding and measuring morbidity; and appropriate measures of the putative causal variables. We shall now look at each of these, paying particular attention to measures of morbidity. To do a survey for its own sake is a blind pursuit, particularly when it will certainly be expensive in valuable manpower which might be better deployed in providing services. Sartorius (1977) has argued powerfully for the need to have research, including surveys, which actually leads to better care of the mentally ill, rather than reiteratively describe patterns of morbidity. The second requirement is a defined population of known size and sociodemographic composition. This is the denominator. It may have geographical boundaries, such as Midtown Manhattan in the well-known study by Srole *et al.* (1962), or the town of Lundby (a pseudonym) in Hagnell's (1966) work. Sometimes it is a population isolate, such as the classic surveys by Strömgren (1938) and later by Fremming (1947) on the island of Bornholm; the study of mental disorders in Iceland by Helgason (1964); or that by Nielsen (1976) in Samsø. The researcher can attempt either to examine all persons in the population, as Hagnell did, or a representative sample of them, which is usually more practicable. There are special techniques for obtaining such a sample, whereby each individual in the population has the same or a known probability of being examined. For such methods, it is wise to consult an experienced survey research worker, and to read in some depth about the principles involved. A good introduction is *Planning and organising a health survey* in the series *Community health surveys* by Lutz (1986).

The strengths of the population survey are that it provides an estimate of how much morbidity is in fact present and is not based only on those cases which reach services; and the study can be extended forward in time to determine outcome. The respective strengths of cross-sectional and cohort studies should be given much thought and attention. The main deficiencies of both are that, compared to case-control studies, surveys are very expensive to conduct; the case-finding has usually to be entrusted to carefully trained lay interviewers; and the yield of cases of some disorders may be low for the effort and cost involved. Some workers are also sceptical about whether the cases identified in a survey are really comparable to clinic cases. Certainly, only a small number of community cases will usually have also found their way to services. The determinants of becoming a case may differ from the determinants of reaching services. Community and clinic cases may differ importantly in severity, in how long the symptoms have persisted, in their social and interpersonal context, and in the amount of social disability associated with them. Standardized methods for assessing morbidity are a keystone of all research in social psychiatry, so we shall now consider this in some detail. Measures of independent variables are discussed in Chapter 4.

CROSS-SECTIONAL AND LONGITUDINAL (COHORT) DESIGNS

We have already noted that a survey may be carried out at only one point in time, when it is said to be cross-sectional. This snapshot shows how the various components are arranged; but it may be limited in revealing how this arrangement came about, although retrospective information may be sought about previous episodes of illness, as well as other relevant social or experiential factors. A better design is *prospective longitudinal*, often called a cohort study, in which the initial sample is re-examined at one or more later points in time. It is then possible to learn more about the circumstances in which some persons became ill, and how others recovered.

INSTRUMENTS FOR MEASURING MORBIDITY

Some discussion is firstly required about the nature of the morbidity we wish to measure. Here the writer has found the thinking of G. A. Foulds (1965) a valuable foundation. In his volume *Personality and personal illness*, Foulds described what he saw as the conceptual boundaries of psychiatric illness, drawing a distinction between this and abnormalities of personality. In this present book, we shall recurrently have to confront this distinction between illness and personality. To Foulds, these were two separate universes of discourse. He saw personality as an assembly of traits and attitudes; and illness as characterized by symptoms and signs. These differ in three important ways (Foulds, 1965, pp. 19–28):

1. Traits and attitudes are universal; symptoms and signs are not. Everyone has the former, but only a few have the latter.
2. Traits and attitudes are relatively ego-syntonic; symptoms and signs are distressful, either to the person or to his or her closest associates.
3. Traits and attitudes are relatively enduring; symptoms and signs tend to fluctuate, or to disappear over time.

Foulds argued that we are all more or less dependent, more or less retiring; but that we do not all have depressive symptoms, delusions or anorexia nervosa. He acknowledged that the distinction is not always simple, because the phenomena are sometimes dimensional, as in the progression from obsessional traits into obsessional symptoms. But in thinking about mental disorders, and in constructing instruments to measure morbidity, we run into difficulties when symptoms and traits are allowed to be mixed together. For example, we may want to measure certain personality traits because they may serve as an index of vulnerability. It will be important to do so without the measure being inflated (contaminated) by symptoms, such as of anxiety or depression. This issue is now a recurrent problem in research on neuroticism or self-esteem as vulnerability factors for depression (see Chapter 4). In what follows, the reader will find it useful to try to make a distinction between illness and personality attributes.

To undertake research in social psychiatry, it is sometimes reasonable to accept the diagnoses made on patients by their doctor. This happens invariably, for example, in case registers. But it is known that clinicians can be seriously unreliable in the diagnoses reached when they are left to their own day-to-day practices, without some restraints in the methods they use. This was demonstrated in a study of fundamental importance by Kreitman (1961). A full exposition is to be found in the important volume by Kendell (1975) on *The role of diagnosis in psychiatry*. For research it is usually necessary to have a more systematic method for determining firstly the likely presence of psychiatric disorder, and secondly what diagnosis can be made. For this, the two main approaches are the questionnaire and the standardized interview.

Psychiatric questionnaires

These are usually quite brief lists of questions which can be handed on a sheet to a patient, or to a respondent in a population survey, for self-completion. If the person is handicapped or unable to read, it may have to be read out. Such questionnaires do not purport to make a diagnosis, but rather to produce a score. On the basis of normative data, this can then be used either as a continuous measure, or a cut-point imposed to divide people into two classes: those likely to be 'cases' according to specified criteria, and those likely not to be. By far the best known instrument of this type in psychiatry is the General Health Questionnaire (GHQ) developed by Goldberg (1972, 1978) and Goldberg and Williams (1988), which has had a profound influence on the progress of research. It can be used in its 60, 30, 28, and 12 item forms. The GHQ was originally developed as a screening instrument to detect persons likely to have a psychiatric disorder in primary care. The 28-item instrument has been factor-analysed to yield separate scores for anxiety and depression (Goldberg and Hillier 1979). For the detection of chronic symptoms, Goodchild and Duncan-Jones (1985) have recommended a modified scoring method, and this seems to be a useful addition. The GHQ does not claim to make a diagnosis, but rather to give a score on a dimension of psychological symptoms; and with appropriate cutting points to determine whether or not a person is likely to be a case of non-psychotic psychiatric disorder. The GHQ can be harnessed to a psychiatric interview in a two-phase design, as developed by Duncan-Jones and Henderson (1978) with the Present State Examination (Wing *et al.* 1974). This can be an economical use of resources when one wants to obtain something approaching a diagnosis in symptomatic persons in a sizeable population sample.

Other instruments of the same general type are the Hopkins Symptom Checklist (Derogatis *et al.* 1974), the Beck Depression Inventory (Beck 1967), the Zung Self-rating Depression Scale (Zung 1965), and the Delusions-Symptoms-Signs Inventory by Bedford and Foulds (1978). The choice of instrument should be made after consulting experienced researchers and clarifying the exact purpose of its use. Often it is wise to use more than one instrument. This provides wider coverage of symptoms and level of severity. It also reduces 'measurement error', which becomes important in recently developed statistical analyses, such as structural equation models. In these, it is assumed that all instruments for measuring, say, depression, carry a certain amount of error, and that the construct of depression is latent and cannot itself be directly observed or measured. If one has several measures of the construct, one is able to calculate a more accurate estimate of it. Examples of such structural equation modelling are the study of substance abuse in adolescents by Newcomb and Bentler (1987); and the contamination of neuroticism by symptoms in the New Zealand study by Fergusson *et al.* (in press).

Psychiatric interviews

No matter how ably a questionnaire is designed, it cannot be a substitute for a psychiatric interview which will yield something approaching a diagnosis according to internationally used criteria. The only exception to this statement would be when one is content to identify persons who have only a high probability of being cases. Progress of fundamental significance for all of psychiatry has been made since the late-1960s in the development of several standardized interviews. They are standardized in that the question asked and the observations on behaviour are not left to the idiosyncrasies of the interviewer. Variability in this can be greatly reduced, though not completely, by trying to ensure that interviewers behave in the same way, wherever in the world the instrument is being used. Inevitably, some differences are likely and this source of variance has to be accepted, and allowed for.

A second source of variability is what symptoms, signs, and clinical history are necessary to make a specific diagnosis. On this, it is possible to have complete concordance by the investigators' agreeing to accept the same set of research diagnostic criteria. Admittedly, there can be difficulties about how clearly these are specified, and how valid is the construct they define. There are two main sets of research diagnostic criteria which have been developed, and which are making a profound impact on psychiatric research. They make it more certain that investigators in different centres are describing the same disorders or syndromes.

The first set of criteria is in the third edition of the *Diagnostic and statistical manual* (DSM–III), and its revision DSM–III-R, of the American Psychiatric Association (1980, 1987). The second is the section on 'Mental, behavioural and developmental disorders' in the forthcoming tenth revision of the *International classification of diseases* (ICD–10) by the World Health Organization. In this, very considerable effort has been made by clinicians and other experts throughout the world to produce a 'common language' for diseases, including mental disorders, wherever they occur. The ICD–10 criteria consist of two parts. The 'Clinical descriptions and diagnostic guidelines' set out the main clinical features, with brief comments on differential diagnosis. They allow flexibility in the number and balance of symptoms, which is appropriate for the busy clinician. The 'Diagnostic criteria for research' are wholly compatible with the 'Clinical descriptions', but are more precise, dogmatic, and restrictive in their instructions.

We have placed emphasis on the importance of diagnostic criteria because these are the only logical starting point for any standardized interview. If it is to be useful, the latter must *service* the criteria, so that diagnoses can be made reliably, both within and between studies. Accounts of possible aetiology, outcome, services used, and response to treatment can be interpreted only if it is clear what disorders are being described.

For standardized interviews, the most widely used are the following:

1. The Present State Examination (PSE) developed by Wing *et al.* (1974). The ninth edition has a shorter version for population surveys and a full version for clinical studies. It has been translated into all the world's major languages and many minor ones. A glossary of terms and guide to its use have been provided and the short version can be taught to non-medical or wholly lay interviewers (Wing *et al.* 1977; Bebbington *et al.* 1981*a*). Ratings are used in the Index of Definition computer algorithm to provide eight levels of likelihood that sufficient symptoms are present to make a classification according to ICD–9. At the threshold level, (5) and above, the CATEGO programme provides a tentative ICD–9 'diagnosis'. The text of the PSE–9 is given in Wing *et al.* (1974), together with the Glossary of Definitions. The instrument itself is set out in a companion booklet (Wing *et al.* 1988). The time-period covered is deliberately restricted to the previous four weeks, because respondents are more likely to report accurately for this compared to a longer time-span. The system is flexible, however, in that ratings can be made separately for the present episode, as well as for the previous four weeks. This distinction is also used in the SCAN (see below). A separate Syndrome Check List can be used for rating previous episodes.

2. The Diagnostic Interview Schedule (DIS) by Robins *et al.* (1981). This instrument was developed for the large Epidemiologic Catchment Area studies in the United States (Regier and Burke, 1988). It is considerably longer than the PSE, covering more syndromes, as defined in the DSM–III. It seeks to determine lifetime prevalence as well as prevalence over recent months. The former is dependent on persons' being able to report episodes long past with the same validity as more recent symptoms. It is unclear if this is achieved. Like the PSE, there is a computer algorithm for generating DSM–III diagnoses.

3. The Composite International Diagnostic Interview (CIDI). This instrument is a combination of the DIS and PSE, and was developed jointly by their authors for the World Health Organization. It can yield both DSM–III diagnoses and be processed by part of the CATEGO-ID system used with the PSE. It is presently undergoing extensive field trials in several countries.

4. The Schedule for Affective Disorders and Schizophrenia (SADS) (Endicott and Spitzer 1978) is a standardized interview which determines the presence of symptoms in these two diagnostic groups. The lifetime version (SADS-L) is the commonest used.

5. The Schedules for Clinical Assessment in Neuropsychiatry (SCAN) are being developed by Wing and his collaborators. This instrument is based on a modular construction and allows diagnoses to be made both by the ICD–10 and DSM–III systems. Modules are being developed to deal with special categories or groups, including dementia, personality disorder or social impairment. The SCAN should be seen as a successor to the PSE.

Interviews by computer

Questionnaires and standardized interviews lend themselves to presentation on a computer screen, the respondent answering by pressing only one or two keys according to some convention; or an interviewer can use the screen as a text, keying in the respondent's replies. In both methods, the result of the interview is available immediately it has ended. Contrary to what might be expected, most people find the procedure very acceptable. Some advantages are that the computer can readily follow branching and cut-offs in the interview, so that the correct sequence of items is always asked; and the responses can be assembled automatically by an algorithm into the equivalent of a diagnosis, or a score on selected scales. The GHQ and most of the standardized interviews described above have each been used in this way. In psychogeriatrics, a number of research groups have now developed neuropsychological tests of considerable sophistication, using a colour visual display unit.

THE CONCEPT OF A CASE

In all that we have discussed so far, it has been implied that the general population can be divided into two distinct groups. First are persons who are ill, whether or not they have reached services. They are usually called 'cases'. The remainder of the population, who are numerically greater, are non-cases. There are times when it is convenient to accept this viewpoint, although it does not reflect the true distribution of morbidity, which is a continuum. This important subject has been extensively examined in the volume *What is a case?*

(Wing *et al.* 1981). A 'case' exists only in a particular context, so that it can be defined as a person reaching psychiatric services, or being recognized as psychologically unwell. But a case can also be defined arbitrarily in a population survey, on the grounds of having a certain level of symptoms, or disability due to them. The cutting point for that has to be decided by the investigators for the purposes in hand. Whereas the concept of a case may be appropriate for clinical work and some research purposes, it is really an artificial dichotomy: most, and possibly all psychiatric syndromes are continual, not categorical or binary states which have to be either present or absent. Some analyses are better conducted on continuous measures rather than on categorical data, since this loses less information and enables the association between the disorder and other variables to be examined more thoroughly. Accordingly, in analysing survey data, scores on dimensional measures should often be considered in addition to examination of attributes only in those who reach case levels of severity. For this, symptom scores for dimensions such as anxiety, depression, and cognitive impairment should be derived in addition, either from the standardized psychiatric interview itself, or from a supplementary instrument. A particular attraction here is the recent application of *latent trait analysis* to psychiatric epidemiology. Among other advantages, this allows the properties of individual items to be examined, according to the level of severity where each item falls on the underlying dimension, and how discriminating each is in separating persons above and below that particular level. An introduction to latent trait analysis has been provided by Duncan-Jones *et al.* (1986). Because of importance in the measurement of morbidity, as well as its considerable heuristic value, a brief overview is given here.

First, it is assumed that the clinical syndromes we wish to examine cannot be observed and measured directly: we can observe only their symptoms, and then infer the presence of an entity such as depression from these. Secondly, each symptom or sign is either present or absent: that is, we impose a binary state on it. Thirdly, the latent trait model is represented in a figure (Fig. 2.2) where the horizontal axis is the latent continuum of, say, depression; and the vertical axis is the probability that a person with a given level of depression will have a particular symptom, or reach the case criteria for, say, major depression in DSM–III-R. Fourthly, each of the symptoms in an interview instrument or questionnaire, represented by items 1, 2, and 3 in Fig. 2.2, is characterized by two properties: its *threshold*, which is how far up the

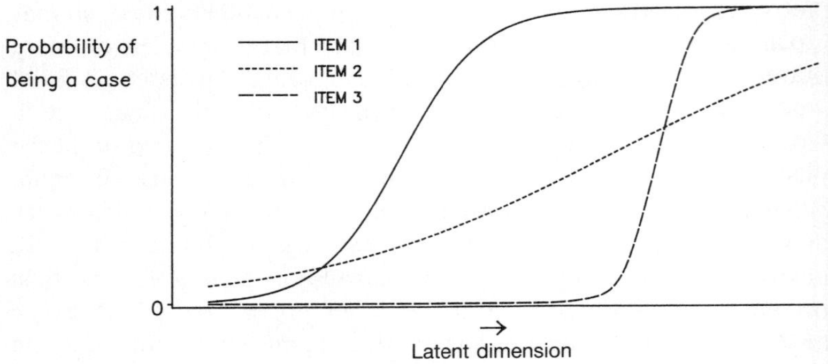

Fig. 2.2. The latent trait model. Three items with contrasted properties.

continuum it lies, where 50 per cent of persons with that level of depression will have that symptom; and its *slope*, which is its discriminating capacity, shown by how steeply the probability of having the symptom increases for a given increment in the level of the disorder. Good items have steep slopes, such as item 3. Items placed low on the continuum, such as item 1, will be more suitable for detecting milder levels of depression, as in general practice or the community; and items towards the right end of the continuum will be relevant to more severe depression, as seen in hospitals (item 3). Item 2 is poor, because it has a weak slope and therefore little discriminatory power: a large increment in severity on the latent dimension is not accompanied by a large increase in the probability of being a case. The latent trait model represents a significant advance for designing better clinical instruments and for analysing them in relation to causal variables. The method has been used on psychiatric interviews in general practice to explore the dimensions of neurosis seen in such settings (Goldberg *et al.* 1987). Using interview data from the Hobart Survey of the Elderly (Kay *et al.* 1985), Grayson *et al.* (1987) were able to determine the properties of items in the Geriatric Mental State and Mini-Mental State Examinations for diagnosing dementia and depression.

THE RANGE OF INDEPENDENT VARIABLES

In social psychiatry, the independent variables are usually some component of the social environment, past or present. They may be aetiological or they may be related to outcome. The simplest of them are sociodemographic, as in age, sex, social class, or marital status. But for more developed hypotheses, experiential variables have to be introduced. These may refer to early life; or to more recent exposure to adversity, and to the social environment around the person. Only rarely have epidemiologists tried to assess personality factors as an index of vulnerability. This is probably because they are difficult to measure validly in a survey setting, despite their likely importance. Psychiatric epidemiologists have also made little progress in the inclusion of biological measures. These usually involve taking a blood sample or other tissue for laboratory examination; or making neurophysiological measures, usually possible only under laboratory conditions. These may be difficult to undertake in population surveys; but it is regrettable on scientific grounds that psychiatric epidemiology has been largely confined to psychosocial variables.

In Chapter 3, we examine how we can organize our thinking about the knowledge already available, or now sought, in social psychiatry, where the various categories of mental disorder are the dependent variables, and where we wish to consider systematically the whole range of independent variables to which they may be related.

Notes

1. Training courses on the DIS and the text of the instrument itself are obtainable from the Department of Psychiatry, Washington University School of Medicine, St. Louis, Missouri 63110, USA (Dr L. N. Robins).

2. The text of the CIDI and training in its use are available from the same centre as for the DIS.

3. The text of the SCAN is available from the MRC Social Psychiatry Unit, Institute of Psychiatry, De Crespigny Park, Denmark Hill, London SE5 8AF, UK (Professor J. K. Wing).

3

Epidemiological knowledge about mental disorders

A matrix for organizing epidemiological knowledge: age, sex, marital status; social class; urbanization; regional variation; secular change; macrosocial and transcultural factors.

A MATRIX FOR ORGANIZING EPIDEMIOLOGICAL KNOWLEDGE

The distribution of mental disorders across the world's population follows a well-defined and remarkably consistent pattern. It is the business of epidemiology to determine this distribution, what factors determine it for particular disorders, and what measures may contribute towards their prevention. For these tasks, as we have already seen, there are four fundamental requirements: a hypothesis, a population (of patients or a community); specification of the psychiatric disorders which are to be investigated; and specification of the set of independent variables which may contribute to their onset or outcome. We shall now use this structure to form a cognitive map. This is useful as a method for organizing in our minds what knowledge is presently available; and for providing a pointer to further avenues of enquiry. This map, which is in the form of a matrix, is conveniently divided into two parts: one for knowledge about aetiology (Table 3.1); and the other for knowledge about services (Table 3.2). We shall look at these in turn.

Knowledge about aetiology

The columns consist of a listing of the main psychiatric disorders. While only general headings are used here, it is clear that a much finer set of categories will be appropriate for other purposes, as for example in considering the epidemiology of childhood psychiatric disorder. The affective and neurotic disorders both need to be further differentiated when we come to consider the dominant factors in their aetiology. Each diagnostic group, furthermore, should not be conceptualized as being frozen in time. Each has its own natural

Table 3.1 A matrix for organizing epidemiological knowledge in psychiatry: aetiology

		CHILD PSYCHIATRIC DISORDERS	NEUROSES	AFFECTIVE DISORDERS	SCHIZOPHRENIA	DEMENTIA	ALCOHOL ABUSE	DRUG ABUSE	SUICIDE	PARASUICIDE	MENTAL RETARDATION	PSYCHOLOGICAL WELL-BEING
SOCIODEMOGRAPHIC FACTORS	Sex											
	Age											
	Marital status											
	Social class											
	Urbanization											
	Regional variation											
	Secular change											
	Other macrosocial factors											
EXPERIENTIAL FACTORS	Seasonality of birth											
	Birth order											
	Parental age											
	Childhood separation											
	Parental style											
	Adverse experiences and events											
	Extreme experiences											
	Bereavement											
	Expressed emotion											
	Unemployment											
	Social support											
	Migration											
	Noise											
	Environmental toxins											
	Dietary factors											
	Personality and temperament											
	Family history											
	Biological factors											
	Interaction of two or more factors											
	Natural history											

history, and it is one of the contributions of epidemiology to determine this. Medicine is currently criticized for being overly concerned with illness, to the neglect of positive health. Readers can therefore consider plausible hypotheses about psychological well-being, as the last entry in the columns.

The rows are provided by those variables which are the postulated causes or modifying factors in psychiatric illnesses. In Table 3.1, these have been arranged into groups: first, sociodemographic and macro-social factors; then experiential factors which befall people during their lifetime. This includes exposures to physical agents, such as infections, environmental toxins, and dietary factors. Another major group in aetiology is in the domain of personality and temperament. This is known to be important, but there is a remarkable lack of epidemiological data on it. Table 3.1 next includes biological vulnerability, including genetic transmission of this. There is then the very real issue of interaction between two or more of any of these variables. This is particularly relevant because mental disorders, perhaps more than many physical diseases, tend to have multiple causes. It is in fact impossible to name a single psychiatric disorder which has only one cause. (Conditions such as Huntington's chorea are taken here to be neurological.) Mental disorders require the occurrence of several factors, and these may each have their point of impact at a different period in a person's lifetime, from the moment of conception. A matter for consideration in its own right is the course or natural history of each diagnostic category, and of factors which influence this. The matrix, it is emphasized, stretches across time.

The reader should at this point study the column and row items, then think about the significance of the cells defined by them. Many of the row variables are to be seen as really having a deeper meaning than their abbreviated label initially implies. This is because of two important features which recur in all epidemiological analyses. The first is *confounding*. An apparently clear-cut variable such as age may be linked to other attributes of the individual, which themselves have an association with mental disorder. For example, in a survey of a population with many elderly persons in it, being old will mean more than being of advanced age: it will *also* mean a greater probability of being female, widowed, having a low income, having impaired physical health, and being less mobile, to mention only some factors typically linked to being elderly. In this way, age may act as a proxy for other social or biological attributes. Such confounding of one factor by others is a problem most of all when it is not recognized by the researcher. The associations then reported are not what they seem to be: the confounding variables may not be contributing to the causes of the disorder.

A second reason for caution in reading the rows is the variability within each experiential variable. For example, it is not enough to consider childhood separation experiences as a homogeneous phenomenon. The significance will be profoundly influenced by other factors, such as the child's age at the time, his temperament, how often it occurred, its permanence, and above all the quality of the care received from others. This illustrates how many of the postulated causal factors can be multi-faceted; and how there is abundant room for variability between individuals, and therefore between studies.

The matrix in Table 3.1 is bulky, but it has heuristic value in that it prompts us to be systematic in assessing the body of knowledge called psychiatric epidemiology; and it leads to further questions emerging in the reader's mind. In some of the cells, is there a need for rather better information? Does it help if categories are defined more specifically in the columns (disorders)? Can new independent variables (rows) be proposed? Has there been undue attention given to some cells in recent research efforts, such as all the work on life-events?

The matrix delineates the present boundaries of knowledge in psychiatric epidemiology and social psychiatry. But most of all, it makes clear what paradigms have been pursued throughout the 20th century. To the present writer, one deficiency has lain in a tendency to explore a particular experiential factor without at the same time considering constitutional vulnerabilities. In this way, psychiatric epidemiology has leant too much on social psychiatry, with relative neglect of the intrapersonal and biological domains.

Knowledge about services

We can go on to construct a matrix for what is known about services for mental disorders (Table 3.2). The columns remain the major categories of psychiatric disorder, as before. The rows refer to the social consequences on the family and community; the proportion of persons in each category who reach primary care or specialist services; the personal and economic burden they bring; social factors related to treatment which epidemiological research may identify;

Table 3.2 A matrix for organizing epidemiological knowledge in psychiatry: services for mental disorders.

		CHILD PSYCHIATRIC DISORDERS	NEUROSES	AFFECTIVE DISORDERS	SCHIZOPHRENIA	DEMENTIA	ALCOHOL OR DRUG ABUSE	SUICIDE	PARASUICIDE	MENTAL RETARDATION	PSYCHOLOGICAL WELL-BEING
	Social consequences: –on the family –on the community										
SERVICES	Proportion reaching primary care										
SERVICES	Proportion reaching psychiatric/specialist services										
SERVICES	Social management or specific treatments										
	Knowledge available for: –primary prevention –secondary prevention –tertiary prevention										
	Evaluation of services										
	Tertiary prevention										

then, in what Gruenberg has called 'the ultimate service of epidemiology', knowledge which can be used for prevention; and finally, the evaluation of services.

Taken together, Tables 3.1 and 3.2 constitute an immense agenda. In the chapters which follow, we shall look selectively at a number of the main issues. Some of the cells have not been tackled, as in epidemiological studies of suicidal behaviour which have been thoroughly described elsewhere (e.g. WHO 1968; Kreitman 1988). Other cells have been omitted because they are irrelevant, at least as far as we know, as in the contribution of unemployment to the onset of dementia. Still others are neglected because little or no information is presently available, despite the legitimacy of the hypothesis, as with dietary factors in any of the psychiatric disorders. What is already known about the epidemiology of psychological well-being (Diener 1984) as the opposite of morbidity, has not been included, although the matrix certainly seems to raise some attractive questions about it, and it is becoming an important social and public health issue. Even with these omissions and blank cells, the remaining agenda is a sizeable one.

We can now consider the principal findings about how psychiatric disorders are distributed in the population. Examining the distribution by age, sex, and other sociodemographic variables is *not* a tedious exercise: it frequently is the start to a train of enquiry into some fundamental factors in aetiology. This is because each of these sociodemographic variables carries with it a number of other factors; that is, it is associated with, or is an indirect expression of, factors which may influence the onset of course of mental disorders. For example, sex or gender is associated with two different biological conditions, two different experiences in earlier life, and two different social roles. Analogous statements can be made about age, marital status, and social class, although there are many more than two conditions for each of these.

In what follows, the reader should bear in mind that we are at times referring to knowledge about mental disorders as they occur in the general population, at others to patients who have come to their general practitioner or a hospital; and at others to the contrast between the two.

AGE, SEX, AND MARITAL STATUS

Children and adolescents

Field surveys have consistently shown that there are differences in the pattern of psychiatric disorders and disabilities between boys and girls; and that the prevalence of these alters with age. Useful reviews of the epidemiology of child and adolescent psychiatric disorders are to be found in Graham (1977), Links (1983), and Rutter and

Sandberg (1985). Here we focus only on age and gender as the independent variables. Lapouse and Monk (1958) examined a community sample of 482 children aged 6 to 12 years and their mothers in Buffalo, New York. Fifty per cent of the girls, but only 36 per cent of the boys had seven or more fears or worries, a statistically significant difference. As in the earlier British study by Blomfield and Douglas (1956), bedwetting was more common in boys: in those aged 6 to 8 years; 8 per cent wet the bed twice or more a week, compared to only 2 per cent of girls. Rutter *et al.* (1973) found that 'pathological' enuresis is found largely over the age of four years, because that is when the spontaneous remission rate plunges. There is an increase in the incidence of enuresis between five and seven years, so that children can gain bladder control then lose it (Rutter and Sandberg 1985).

Some of the most comprehensive information on the epidemiology of childhood and adolescent mental disorders has come from field studies in the Isle of Wight and London by Rutter and his colleagues (Rutter *et al.* 1976). Emotional disorders were found to be slightly more common in girls, whereas behaviour and conduct disorders occurred more in boys. By the mid-teens, psychiatric disorders were twice as common in boys, due entirely to the higher rate of conduct and mixed disorders. In 14 and 15 year olds in the Isle of Wight study, emotional disorders *per se* were equally common in the two sexes.

Adult neurosis and affective disorder

In adults the prevalence of minor psychiatric disorders, particularly anxiety and depression, is consistently found to be higher in women, sometimes by as much as two-fold. The sex difference is usually greatest between 20 and 45 years. This holds for most studies in Western industrialized countries. In the recent Epidemiologic Catchment Area (ECA) studies in three US cities (Robins *et al.* 1984), the lifetime prevalence of major depression, dysthymia, and phobic states was appreciably higher in women. A notable finding has been that, although the six-month prevalence of major depression is more frequent in women (2·4 : 1), the sex ratio for bipolar disorder is about equal (Weissman *et al.* 1984).

This female excess in morbidity occurs both in field surveys and in persons reaching services, including primary care. It does not seem to be due to biased case-ascertainment, as might occur if the instruments contained items which women were more likely to endorse, even if they were mentally healthy; or if doctors were sexually biased in diagnosing neurotic or affective disorders. The sex difference is now accepted by most as real. This poses a major challenge for its explanation. Weissman and Klerman (1977) made a careful analysis of the possibilities for depression. There could be greater biological susceptibility in women; or psychosocial factors could act to induce depression more in them than in men. In the biological domain, consideration has been given to a possible effect from genes on the X chromosome; or to some consequence of female reproductive physiology, particularly in the endocrine system. In the psychosocial domain, two hypotheses are favoured: the social status of women; and learned helplessness.

As Weissman and Klerman emphasize, it is unlikely that any single factor accounts for all of the sex difference in rates. Investigators have unfortunately tended to focus on only one domain, such as the biological or social role hypotheses, without taking account of the work in other disciplines. A finding which lends credence to the social status and role of women as one powerful factor is the evidence suggesting that marriage is protective for men but detrimental for women, at least in relation to depressive disorders (Bebbington *et al.* 1981*a*; Der and Bebbington 1987; Bebbington 1987*a*, 1988). Tennant (1985*a*) has written a succinct critique of the evidence for female vulnerability to depression, concluding that social risk factors probably act independently of each other, and that these may vary considerably between populations of women. This latter point may be highly relevant in interpreting discordant findings on the causal role of life-events or social support, because these may be acting on groups with different vulnerabilities. A considerable literature has now grown on the possible reasons for sex differences in the incidence of minor psychiatric disorder. For a recent account, with useful bibliographies, the reader is referred to the concise monographs by Briscoe (1982) and Jenkins (1985). Jenkins concluded from her own study that there is a sex difference in the consultation of general practitioners and in the consumption of prescribed non-psychotropic medication by individuals with minor psychiatric symptoms; but she found no evidence that women assess their own health differently. It does appear that women are more likely than men to express their emotional difficulties (Briscoe 1982). This is thought to be due to underlying biological and/or social factors. Briscoe concluded that: 'sex differences in minor psychiatric morbidity are not primarily due to varying pathological influences (such as role strain) or to extraneous factors (such as physician bias or time constraints) but rather reflect basic sociopsychological differences in masculinity and femininity'.

The relationship of age to the incidence or prevalence of affective disorder and neurosis makes an untidy story. *Unipolar depression* has a much later age of onset than the *bipolar form*, where Clayton (1981) found the average age of onset to be about 30 years. By the age of 50 years, 90 per cent of bipolar cases have been diagnosed, in contrast to the unipolar form where the age of first onset tends to be in the second half of life. Bebbington *et al.* (1981*b*) reviewed the findings on minor psychiatric disorder in earlier surveys of general populations, concluding that no clear pattern emerged. In their own Camberwell study, they found no change with age in prevalence for men, but two peaks at 25–34 and 45–54 for women. In the ECA studies (Robins *et al.* 1984), dysthymic disorder, taken here to be the equivalent of neurotic depression, did not show any consistent change in frequency with age.

The implication of these findings for clinical practice is that anxiety and some other neurotic disorders do become less frequent with age. The emergence of such conditions for the first time in the second half of life is atypical and should prompt a thorough search for causes. It is unclear why the first half of adult life should be accompanied by more anxiety and depressive disorders. It may be that child-raising, occupational pressures, and age-related difficulties in personal relationships bring their stressor effects; or that older adults are less emotionally reactive, having acquired more effective coping mechanisms. These are fundamental issues, although ones in which social psychiatry has yet to produce conclusive evidence.

Schizophrenia

The age-specific incidence of treated schizophrenia is significantly earlier in men than in women. This is a consistent finding, described by Eaton (1985) in his comprehensive review of its epidemiology. Males have a peak incidence at 15–24 years, but women at 25–34 years. This 10-year difference could have been induced artifactually if men reached treatment earlier, because the incidence data are derived from hospitals or clinics and do not refer to the emergence of new cases in the general population. But there is evidence against this from community data, suggesting that the age and sex difference is real. The cause of it is unknown.

Marital status At the time of onset of schizophrenia, more persons are unmarried than would be expected from the general population. This has been repeatedly confirmed and suggests a selection effect, whereby persons who develop schizophrenia are less likely to have previously established a marital relationship, or to have maintained it (Susser *et al.* 1970*a,b*; Eaton 1985).

Alcohol abuse

The epidemiology of alcohol abuse presents a number of difficulties peculiar to the syndrome and its associated behaviours. These have to be considered before looking at the sociodemographic distribution of alcohol-related problems. Good accounts of the subject have been provided by Kreitman (1977*a*), Edwards (1980), and Chick (1982). The main difficulties are: (1) criterion variation in diagnosing cases; (2) uncertainty about the relationship between different indices of abuse; (3) limitations of the household survey method for case-detection; and (4) limitations of data about consumption obtained by self-report.

Alcohol abuse is very much a dimensional condition, so that there is no absolute cutting-point between cases and non-cases. Indeed, an adequate clinical definition of the alcohol dependence syndrome has proved difficult to develop (Edwards and Gross 1976; Edwards 1980). The main indicators of alcohol abuse are hospital admission rates, deaths from cirrhosis, deaths from alcoholism, offences of drunkenness, national or regional per capita consumption and, lastly, estimates made in community surveys of personal consumption and of alcohol-related problems. The relationship between these can be complicated, as in the debate concerning national consumption and how this relates to the proportion of the population who become cases (Bruun *et al.* 1975).

In community surveys, it is likely that some of those who are not contacted and interviewed have some alcohol-related difficulties. When an interview is accomplished, it is well-established that heavy drinkers under-report their intake, although interview by computer has now been shown to improve this considerably (Lucas *et al.* 1977; Ogden 1983). Standardized questionnaires, either for self-completion or interview use, have a number of deficiencies, including a variable time-reference. There has been debate about whether it is better to use a diary method, in which the respondent reports what alcohol has been consumed each day for the previous week or more; or whether he should he asked to report his usual consumption over a longer period. It seems clear that the best approach is to take a standardized history of all activities, including drinking, over a specified period in the immediate past. This will generate more accurate information than questionnaires such as the MAST. Biological tests such as γ-glutamyl transferase and mean cell volume are related only to recent consumption. The use of informants for detecting alcohol abuse has not been found to bring a gain in information as much as in some other disorders.

Despite all these difficulties, some clear sociodemographic trends do exist. Whenever alcohol is used in the world, men drink considerably more than women; and there are more cases of alcohol dependency amongst them. Younger adults are now the heaviest consumers in many countries. Age-specific rates indicate that many men reduce their intake as they age or marry. Drew (1968) concluded that the prevalence of treated cases of alcoholism diminishes more rapidly with age than can be explained by successful treatment or mortality; some appear to grow out of it in later adulthood. For marital status, there is a definite excess of single, separated and divorced persons of both sexes. Co-morbidity with alcohol abuse is very considerable and extends across the physical, mental, and social domains. Malignant, respiratory, and cardiovascular diseases, depression, suicide, and antisocial behaviour number prominently amongst these.

Dementia

The prevalence of both presenile and senile dementia of Alzheimer type (SDAT) is probably higher in women, according to a meta-analysis of 27 studies by Jorm *et al.* (1987). For vascular or multi-infarct dementia (MID), there is some excess of males, probably related to more hypertension and vascular disease. The incidence of the dementias increases steeply with age from the seventh decade of life. Age-specific incidence rates for a total population have been reported for both the main types, senile and vascular dementia, by Hagnell *et al.* (1981, 1983). The prevalence of all dementias is estimated to be about 0·7 per cent of persons aged 60–64 years, but as much as 38·6 per cent in those aged 90 years and over (Jorm *et al.* 1987). This increase in prevalence is due to two factors. First, there is the steep rise in the age-specific incidence. Secondly, dementia is a chronic disorder, so that incident cases lead to an accumulating prevalence with increasing age. Furthermore, this century has seen an increase in the survival of persons with chronic diseases. Gruenberg (1977) has drawn attention to this phenomenon for cases of dementia and other chronic disabilities. It is probably attributable in large part to more effective medical care. He has wryly called it 'the failures of success'. Gruenberg *et al.* (1976) expressed it pointedly: 'The old man's friend, pneumonia, is dead—a victim of medical progress'.

Some workers have raised the possibility that there is a plateau in the incidence after about 80 years (Jarvik *et al.* 1980), whereby if a person reaches that age and has not yet developed a dementia, the subsequent risk is much lower. This attractive proposition has yet to be confirmed in a general population sample. It has not been supported by Hagnell's findings on age-specific incidence (Hagnell *et al.* 1981, 1983; Rorsman *et al.* 1985; Henderson 1986).

Age of onset There has been some confusion about the relationship of Alzheimer's disease (a presenile disorder) to senile dementia. Amaducci *et al.* (1986) have assembled interesting historical information on how this arose. The prevailing belief now is that it is the same disorder, but there may be at least two types, in which age of onset is one distinguishing feature. Type 1 is of later onset, usually after the age of 65 years. It is typically slow in progression and memory impairment is conspicuous. Type 2 usually starts earlier than 65 years, is more rapid and shows temporal-parietal and/or frontal lobe involvement, in addition to memory impairment from hippocampal damage. A family history of similar dementia is more frequent in Type 2. The different ages of onset may be a pointer to different weighting amongst the aetiological factors.

Eating disorders

Anorexia nervosa and bulimia are well known to have their highest incidence in younger women. While admittedly there may be important selection effects in who reaches psychiatric care for a condition which is indisputably dimensional in character, the best epidemiological information on anorexia which is available comes from case registers and surveys of young women in particular settings. Kendell *et al.* (1973) used the psychiatric case registers in Aberdeen, Camberwell, and Monroe County. They found an overwhelming predominance of females, with an average age at first contact between 21 and 24 years. It is likely that a similar pattern holds for bulimia. There are some indications that the age at onset in anorexia nervosa may have dropped in the last two to three decades, possibly in parallel with the secular trend in maturation. It is not uncommon now for the disorder to present in general practice in the mid- or early-teens. The age and sex distribution, together with a striking secular change in incidence, are compatible with an aetiology based largely on social learning, with particular personality traits and family patterns conferring increased susceptibility. That is, girls may have abnormal eating patterns induced through prevalent social attitudes and concepts of what is desirable, as promoted by the advertising industry. Such patterns may be adopted with particular readiness by young girls with certain premorbid personality traits, such as fragile self-esteem and a need for mastery. These propositions, though, are wholly speculative.

Suicide and parasuicide

The incidence of suicide and parasuicide examined by age, sex and marital status follows a particularly well-defined pattern. For a review of their epidemiology, readers are referred to the account by Kreitman (1988), the edited volume on parasuicide by Kreitman (1977*b*) and the publication of the World Health Organization (1982*a*) *Changing patterns in suicide behaviour*. Suicide ranks among the 10 most frequent causes of death in most developed countries. Ascertainment of death by suicide is always underestimated and is dependent on the returns made on death certificates. The suicide rate increases with age in both sexes, being about two times higher in men than women. Since about 1960, the rate for young adults has increased in both sexes in many countries. In Sainsbury's words, (1986, p. 23) this increase provides 'an objective and poignant indication of the predicament of young people today'. Marital status has a marked association with suicide, the rate being highest in the divorced, followed by the single and widowed.

By contrast, parasuicide (attempted suicide) is most common in persons aged 15–25, declining steeply thereafter. Particularly in the young, women have higher rates than men. Like suicide, the divorced carry the highest rates.

SOCIAL CLASS

Social class is an elaborate construct, but it is important for clinicians and epidemiologists to have some understanding of what is done when individuals are so stratified; and what the significance is when such stratification is related to patterns of disease. A useful account of social class or stratification is given in Volume 15 of the *International encyclopedia of the social sciences* (Sills 1968, p. 288). The analogy has been brought from the earth sciences. Stratification implies evaluation of individuals or groups on a scale of values. These include the dimensions of power, occupational prestige, income or wealth, education and knowledge, religious purity (as in India), family or ethnic group position, and local community status. Separately or conjointly, these factors may be related to the incidence of psychiatric disorders, so that asking about the distribution of morbidity in social class is a reasonable question in an epidemiological analysis.

If a disorder occurs more often in one social class, this can be an important lead to aetiology. Typically in medical epidemiology, it may point to exposures or living conditions which favour the development of a disorder. This may lead to a *social causation, or breeder hypothesis*, or to a search for some environmental toxin. In psychiatry, however, and sometimes in general medicine, there is often an alternative interpretation to entertain, because people's behaviour may act as an intervening variable for a causal process running in the reverse direction: the disorder itself or its prodromata may alter behaviour in a way which leads to a change in social class. This is a *social selection or drift hypothesis*. Both the breeder and drift hypotheses hold considerable intellectual and political appeal, and both have fuelled intensive research by social scientists. Either hypothesis is much improved if it is referred to a specific psychiatric disorder, rather than being generally applied to all forms of psychiatric morbidity. One has to be wary of an artifact in the rates found for different classes: there may be different thresholds operating in the minds of those making a diagnosis. That is, the diagnosis of, say, schizophrenia or dementia, may be made more often in persons from the most disadvantaged class.

Neurotic and affective disorders

Dohrenwend and Dohrenwend (1969) carried out a searching review of the literature to conclude that, for neurosis, the highest rates were reported about equally often in the lowest social class and in some other class. Boyd and Weissman (1981) have noted an inverse relationship between depressive symptoms and social class in several field studies. On the other hand, where fairly homogeneous populations have been studied, no association has emerged between social class and depression (Taylor and Chave 1964; Hare and Shaw 1965; Brown and Harris 1978). Hagnell (1966) found no difference in the incidence of such mental disorders in those earning under or over 6000 Swedish kröner a year. In the second Camberwell study, Bebbington *et al.* (1981*a*) found only a trend towards higher prevalence rates in working class men and women. They did find a small but significant negative correlation between total PSE score and social class. In Canberra, no association was found between minor morbidity and social class (Henderson *et al.* 1981).

The Epidemiologic Catchment Area studies in the United States, based on very large samples with a wide spread of social class within and between centres, examined education and prevalence to find that, overall, those with a college (tertiary) education had lower rates for anxiety disorders, including phobias, but no statistically significant difference for either major depression or dysthymia (Robins *et al.* 1984).

Studies of non-Western populations show a similar trend, with an inverse association between general psychiatric morbidity and social class or education. In their field survey of a village in Karnataka State, India, Carstairs and Kapur (1976) found higher rates for minor psychiatric disorder in men and women with limited education. When rates were compared across three castes, the Brahmins had lower rates than either Bants (farmers) or Mogers (fishermen), although the differences were not striking. High case rates were found in women, but not men, who had changed over from a traditional, matrilineal pattern of residence after their marriage to living with their husbands' family.

There is some evidence that *mania* and *bipolar disorder* may be over-represented in social class 1 and 2 (Bagley, 1973), although Bebbington (1988) did not find this in his examination of admission rates. Bagley has suggested that the excess in the upper social class could be a diagnostic artifact; or that manic-depressive disorder is associated with an energetic personality which favours a rise in social class (a drift hypothesis); or that the pressures of upper class life, and of having risen there, may contribute to the onset (a breeder hypothesis). There is no conclusive evidence on this, and the subject has not been investigated as thoroughly as for schizophrenia.

Conclusion Where there is indeed a steep gradient in living conditions, whereby the lowest social class carries a substantially higher burden of adversity, higher rates for neurosis and depressive disorders may exist. In some population groups, such as working class women in London, the rates for depression have been found to be very high indeed (Brown and Harris 1978). But in most major surveys, including the large ECA data set, no clear gradient has been demonstrated.

Schizophrenia

Neither the incidence nor the prevalence of schizophrenia are randomly distributed across the social classes. Consistently, more cases are found in the lowest class than would be expected by chance. Dohrenwend and Dohrenwend (1969) listed seven surveys in which estimates of the prevalence of schizophrenia had been made. These included point prevalence, lifetime rates, and treated prevalence. Five showed the highest rates in the lowest social class. Eaton (1985) looked at the incidence of treated cases, finding that 15 of 17 studies reported the highest rate in the lowest class. The recent ECA studies have again reported the same pattern for lifetime prevalence at the community level, although the difference between college graduates and others reached statistical significance in only one of three sites (Robins *et al.* 1984).

With the increased rates in the lowest social class now firmly established, there has been intense interest in finding an explanation, since this could provide a clue to aetiology. In a particularly thorough review of the epidemiology of schizophrenia, Eaton (1985) has examined the likely explanations of these consistent observations. As foreshadowed at the beginning of this section two competing hypotheses have traditionally been put forward, each implying a different direction of causality. The *breeder hypothesis* proposes that there are factors in the lowest social class which increase the risk for developing schizophrenia: a greater level of adversity, poorer social support, poorer maternal and obstetric care leading to foetal damage (Pasamanick and Knobloch 1966), or increased exposure to infectious diseases or environmental agents. This hypothesis implies that the afflicted individual is already in the lowest social class and experiences the pathogenic exposure at some stage after conception. A direct genetic explanation, invoking the notion of a pool of genes for schizophrenia in the lowest social class, is also credible, although it is difficult to understand how this could have been maintained over many centuries, because in fertility schizophrenia has been appreciably less than the average until recently. It is now said to be the same as the general population.

An alternative explanation is that having schizophrenia or its prodromata leads to a drop in social class, due to inability to function at the social class level of origin, or to progress upwards. This is the *selection or drift hypothesis* and has two versions, as pointed out by Eaton (1985): if the social class mobility is seen as a comparison between parents and afflicted offspring, the mobility is intergenerational. If the comparison is made longitudinally over the individual's own career, the mobility is intra-generational.

There is strong evidence to support the selection or drift hypothesis, particularly in its intergenerational form. In a methodologically elegant study, E. Goldberg and Morrison (1963) produced evidence of considerable significance. They drew a sample of 353 men admitted to mental hospitals in England and Wales and given a diagnosis of schizophrenia. These patients were aged 25–34 years at the time of admission and therefore past the normal age of vocational training. They could be presumed to have reached a reasonably 'final' occupational status. Goldberg and Morrison then compared their social class distribution with the most recent census; and with the distribution of their fathers at the time of the patients' birth. They confirmed the excess of cases in social class 5, but found that the distribution for fathers' social class was the same as the general population. They justifiably concluded that there had therefore been a downwards drift in social class. In New York, Turner and Wagenfeld (1967) showed that there was less upward mobility in social class amongst persons developing schizophrenia. In interpreting either study, there is no evidence to support the view that lower social class persons might be more likely to receive an erroneous diagnosis of schizophrenia. Indeed, Goldberg and Morrison took steps to confirm the diagnoses in their sample, lest such a bias might prove misleading. These findings lend strong support to the selection or drift hypothesis. Using the Aberdeen Psychiatric Case Register, Birtchnell (1971) showed that psychiatric patients were significantly more downwardly mobile than the general population. The social mobility of neurotic patients was similar to the latter, but all other groups showed varying degrees of downwards mobility, this being most extreme in the psychotics.

The conclusion must be that schizophrenia impairs the functioning of individuals, making it more difficult for them to hold the social class of their origin, particularly where the disorder is chronic or frequently recurrent. They therefore tend to decline in social class. As a further point against the breeder hypothesis, it should be borne in mind that working class life in many developing countries carries with it a far harsher life-style than in Western working class conditions, with more severe and more frequent adversity, and a greater probability of exposure to hazards in the environment. Yet, as far as is known, the incidence of schizophrenia is not higher in such countries; and the prognosis is in fact often more favourable (WHO 1979; Sartorius *et al.* 1986; see also p. 150).

Alcohol dependence

There is some evidence for a weak inverse association between alcohol-related problems and social class. There are also high rates in specific occupations. Plant (1978) has discussed this association and its possible causes. Occupations which carry a high risk include the following: brewers and distillery workers; the hotel industry; jobs where the consumption of alcohol is part of the routine with colleagues or clients; and occupations involving atypical living conditions, as with seamen and oil-rig workers. Access to cheap or free drinks places people at risk, as with managing directors, who are known to have high rates. Diplomats, who have access to duty-free alcohol and in whom alcohol consumption is part of working life, could be expected also to have high rates, although details are not available.

The Epidemiologic Catchment Area studies in the United States found no statistically significant difference between college graduates and others in Baltimore and St. Louis, but in New Haven, a higher rate in non-graduates reached the 5 per cent significance level. Rather than examining social class, attention would be better accorded to specific occupations, their social environment, and factors influencing recruitment to them. This approach has been used in Edinburgh by the MRC Unit for Epidemiological Studies in Psychiatry (Kreitman, 1977*a*, 1986).

Dementia

If sound evidence for a non-random distribution of dementia by social class were established, this would be a promising aetiological lead. As there is an urgent need for such clues, particularly for senile dementia of Alzheimer type (SDAT), the question has now become highly relevant. A skew in the social class distribution might suggest some differential exposure to an environmental agent or infection; that is, a breeder hypotheses. One serious problem has so far hindered progress in this: by the very nature of the disorder, cases of dementia may not be uniformly ascertained across social class. Because tests for cognitive impairment are highly dependent on education and intelligence, and because the lowest social class has more persons of limited ability or performance in these respects, the apparent case rate is likely to be higher in the lowest class. Where diagnosis is made by clinical judgement, it again seems likely that more persons in the lowest social class will be diagnosed as demented, even by experienced clinicians. What is uncertain is whether the excess, identified either by cognitive tests or clinical judgement, is an artefact attributable to the ascertainment procedure and educational bias in the tests and in the clinician, or whether it is a real difference.

Bergmann *et al.* (1971) re-assessed between two and four years later the 19 persons ascertained by them in a community survey as likely to have a mild or questionable dementia. Only six had progressed to definite dementia. The remaining persons were thought to have had limited intelligence and education. Bergmann and his colleagues therefore emphasized the dangers of mistaken diagnosis of mild dementia in such social groups.

In the US–UK Cross-National Study of the Elderly in New York and London, Gurland *et al.* (1983) found substantially higher rates for dementia in persons with low education. High scores for dementia were 2·5 times more frequent in the low education group. Importantly, these authors took account of the well-known confounding of educational level by age: because of secular changes, older people will have had fewer educational opportunities. Therefore, the existence of an association between dementia and low education should be looked for *within* age-groups. Gurland and his colleagues found that it persisted. Here, dementia was ascertained mainly by performance on the Mental Status Questionnaire (MSQ) of Kahn *et al.* (1960) . In the so-called *Mini-Finland study*, with a national population sample of 8000 adults, Sulkava *et al.* (1985) found a social class gradient for clinically diagnosed cases of SDAT, the lowest class having higher rates.

In the Epidemiologic Catchment Area studies in the United States, the association has again been demonstrated, although here the instrument was only the Mini-Mental State Examination (MMSE) of Folstein *et al.* (1975), rather than a clinical diagnosis of a specific dementia. In Baltimore and New Haven, a high proportion of persons with cognitive impairment was found in the less educated. Kramer *et al.* (1985) reported that amongst the elderly of East Baltimore with less than six years of education, 12·5 per cent had an MMSE score of under 18, which is taken to indicate severe cognitive impairment. Amongst those with 12 or more years of education, the rate was only 1·6 per cent. There were no significant differences between males and females, or whites and non-whites, specific for educational level. In New Haven, Weissman *et al.* (1985) reported a 30-fold difference in the prevalence of severe cognitive impairment, also ascertained by the MMSE, between those with eight or fewer years of education and those with 16 or more years (6·1 and 0·2 per cent).

These differences call for further exploration. Possible interpretations are: (1) the excess prevalence is an artefact due to biased ascertainment procedures, whether these be cognitive tests such as the MSQ or MMSE, or clinical judgement; (2) the excess is real and is due to a lower threshold for the manifestation of severe cognitive impairment in those with lower education or lower intelligence, or possibly lower neuronal reserves; or (3) the excess is real and is due to higher exposure to pathogenic factors.

These are hypotheses which can now be tested. Until there is a biological test for SDAT, what is needed are research diagnostic criteria and a standardized examination, including a history, which are both as free as possible of the influence of education and premorbid intelligence. Such case-finding will also have to be for specific types of dementia, not just severe cognitive impairment without further differentiation. Because prevalence is affected by the duration of survival, the ideal aim must be to determine the social class distribution of the incidence of SDAT.

URBANIZATION

Urbanization is a useful sociodemographic variable because it may lead to identifying conditions which jeopardize, or indeed promote, health. These could lie in the social or physical environment. In a series of scholarly publications Boyden (1969, 1972, 1980, 1987) has considered the health implications of changes in the social and physical conditions of human settlements during the species' evolution; and the psychosocial accompaniments of the urban environment, an environment which is a very recent arrival in evolutionary terms, and which is markedly different from the savanna environment of hunters and gatherers in which the human biogram developed.

For adults in the late-20th century, urban living conditions may plausibly bring more life stress than rural environments. As life stress is thought to contribute to the onset of both anxiety and depressive disorders, higher rates might be expected in cities than in the countryside. On the other hand, it could be argued that rural communities are more rigid, less tolerant of eccentricity, and understimulating; many rural workers and their families are faced with monotonous toil and fewer leisure opportunities. In either event, selective migration might deplete rural areas of more energetic, upwardly mobile persons, leaving a residue who may have fewer coping resources.

There have been few opportunities to test these hypotheses directly. Rates for treated cases, such as case-registers generate, are unhelpful because of the likelihood of differential access to services. Comparison of urban and rural rates *between* population surveys is unsatisfactory, because differences in the design and case-finding methods may be more than sufficient to explain any differences in the observed prevalence rates. Furthermore, there is no reason to accept that a particular urban or rural area in one country is representative of all urban or rural communities. Both are likely to vary considerably in the strength of those attributes which may influence mental health. We have already seen that a consideration of general mental health is usually unhelpful compared to examination of specific diagnostic categories, so that studies reporting scores on some general scale in urban and rural populations are of limited value. Lastly, when urban versus rural domicile is examined as a binary variable, there may be important confounding effects. If there are more elderly in the rural sample, the attribute 'rural' then becomes a proxy for age. Educational experience may likewise differ systematically. One should also determine whether the urban and rural samples included institutions such as hospitals, nursing homes, special schools, and prisons. The presence of these in one area may increase its prevalence rates. On the other hand, if they are not included, persons in them who have come from the community being studied will be omitted from ascertainment, thereby clouding what can be concluded from the comparison.

The central question in the present context is how specified mental disorders are distributed between rural and urban areas. Their prevalence might also vary *within* cities, according to the characteristics of the suburb or proximity to the central area, as explored in the classical studies of Faris and Dunham (1939). Where such a non-random distribution occurs, there may be three explanations: the environment has some effect on the incidence of the disorder; having the disorder or its prodromata influences where people live; or a third set of factors leads both to the disorder and to the person's area of residence. In the latter two models, it is implied that selective migration has taken place.

Urbanization and psychiatric disorders in childhood

The epidemiological studies of Rutter and his colleagues have allowed a comparison of child psychiatric disorder and specific reading retardation in an urban and rural sample, using the same age-range, the same methods and the same measures in the hands of the same investigators (Rutter *et al.* 1975*a*; Rutter 1981). They compared 10-year-old children in Inner London and the Isle of Wight. Psychiatric morbidity and specific reading retardation were both found to be twice as common in London; and this difference was real, not being attributable to different case-finding methods. It was next shown that the correlates of morbidity were themselves more common in London and were therefore likely factors in explaining the difference. These factors were family disturbance, parental deviance, social disadvantage, and school difficulties (Rutter *et al.* 1975*b*). When morbidity rates in London and the Isle of Wight were standardized for these factors, the area difference disappeared. This showed that the greater morbidity among children in London was attributable to greater adversity in both family and school. Rutter and his colleagues concluded that child psychiatric disorder is related to community influences and social environment conditions as well as to personal and constitutional factors. It may also be proposed from these findings that life in smaller communities somehow protects against psychiatric disorders. Furthermore, as in most other comparisons of urban and rural populations, it is conceivable that selective migration may have contributed to the distribution of morbidity, persons with risk factors being more likely to move to an urban environment.

Urbanization and adult psychiatric disorders

In one of the early classic surveys in psychiatric epidemiology, Tsung-yi Lin and his colleagues compared prevalence rates for specific categories of disorder in urban and rural communities in Taiwan (Lin 1953). He found that there was little difference in the total morbidity rates for an urban area, a small town and a rural area. But rates for mental retardation and senile psychosis were somewhat higher in the rural area, whereas neurosis and psychopathic disorder were more common in the city.

There have been few studies since then, where the same investigators have used the same methods on comparable urban and rural samples. The studies by Rutter and his colleagues compared the prevalence of maternal psychiatric disorder in the Isle of Wight and in London, finding higher rates in the latter. Brown *et al.* (1977) and Brown and Harris (1978) contrasted rates for psychiatric disorder, but also social conditions, in women in the island of North Uist in the Outer Hebrides of Scotland, with women in Inner London. They found three-month prevalence rates for borderline or higher level psychiatric disorder of 24 per cent in North Uist and 33 per cent in Camberwell. Depression was more common in Camberwell, but anxiety and phobic states in North Uist. In that island, psychiatric disorder was unrelated to social class and to having young children at home, in contrast to London. An interesting study by Vazquez Barquero *et al.* (1982) in the northern Spanish province of Navarre found substantially higher rates for neurosis in an 'urban' area (made up of four villages), compared to a 'rural' and an 'isolated' area.

As part of the Epidemiologic Catchment Area studies, Blazer *et al.* (1985) surveyed a total urban and rural sample of nearly 4000 adults. Case-ascertainment was by the Diagnostic Interview Schedule including the Mini-Mental State Examination. Starting with six-month prevalence rates without correction for major confounding variables, they found higher rates in the urban sample for major depression and drug abuse. The rural area had higher rates for alcohol abuse and for cognitive defect in its elderly. Dysthymic disorder, schizophrenia, obsessive-compulsive disorder, antisocial personality, and agoraphobia did not differ. They then used a logistic regression model to control on confounding demographic variables. The finding was that the odds ratio for major depression was nearly twice as high in the urban sample. No disorder was more common in the rural area after this correction. There is no obvious explanation for the urban excess of major depression.

In their meta-analysis of 47 studies of the prevalence of dementia, Jorm *et al.* (1987) found three studies which provided data on rural communities (Jensen 1963; Nielsen 1962; Åkesson 1969). All had significantly lower rates than for urban populations in Scandinavia. This could be an important pointer to differential exposure.

REGIONAL VARIATION

If a psychiatric disorder is found to occur at different rates in different geographic areas, this may be because: (1) it is an artefact due to different methods in constructing the samples, or in case-ascertainment; (2) there are genetic differences conferring different susceptibility; (3) the populations have been exposed to different experiences in the physical or social environment. Comparison of disease rates in different communities has a well-established history for disorders such as coronary heart disease, specific cancers, and disorders of unknown aetiology such as multiple sclerosis. For mental disorders, three groups have received most attention: schizophrenia, dementia, and alcohol abuse.

Schizophrenia

In his review of the epidemiology of schizophrenia, Eaton (1985) reports that two populations have been found to have prevalence rates which are twice as high as others. These are on the Istrian peninsula of Yugoslavia and in the Irish Republic. To these, one should add northern Sweden, in the light of studies by Böök (1953) and Böök *et al.* (1978). A comprehensive review of the general epidemiology of schizophrenia has been set out by Hare (1987).

There had been a longstanding belief by Yugoslav psychiatrists that the prevalence of schizophrenia was higher than elsewhere in the area around the northern end of the Adriatic known as the Istrian peninsula. In a series of steps, a team of Yugoslav and American investigators obtained data to test this hypothesis (Crocetti *et al.* 1971; Lemkau *et al.* 1980). First, a study of hospitalized patients showed an excess of schizophrenia in the Istrian study area compared to Zagreb, though other psychoses were also present in excess. To examine the possibility that this difference was only for treated illnesses, a community survey was conducted both in the Istrian peninsula and elsewhere in Yugoslavia. A higher prevalence of functional psychoses, both schizophrenia and manic-depressive disorder, was found in the Istrian peninsula and the northern Adriatic littoral compared to the rest of Croatia. The difference was not uniform over the population but was most marked in those over 40 years, particularly women. It was not related to educational level, inland or coastal residence, or occupational group. Cigarette smoking was noted to be higher in the study area, but cases did not smoke more than non-cases. Three other disorders were found also to be more common: diabetes mellitus, psoriasis, and alcoholism. The authors concluded that they had succeeded in demonstrating a geographic difference in rates for psychosis, that they had not identified any demonstrable explanation, and that the populations studied offer an opportunity to test both genetic and ecological theories about the aetiology of the functional psychoses.

The increased prevalence of treated schizophrenia in Eire has been much debated (Walsh and Walsh 1970; Scheper-Hughes 1979; Walsh *et al.* 1980; Nuallain *et al.* 1984). The prevalence was found to be as much as double the rates in the United Kingdom. The most likely explanation was that Irish psychiatrists were diagnosing schizophrenia too readily, thereby increasing the officially recorded rates through an artefact in their clinical practice. But recent work, including rating of videotapes by Irish and UK psychiatrists, makes this interpretation unlikely (Kelleher and Copeland 1973, 1974). Walsh *et al.* (1980) attribute it to cultural characteristics influencing treatment patterns, to a higher incidence of schizophrenia, or to a longer course of the illness. Nuallain *et al.* (1984) suggest that an increased incidence, if it exists, is insufficient to explain the higher treated prevalence.

For northern Sweden, Böök *et al.* (1978) confirmed the earlier finding of increased prevalence (Böök 1953). The rate was three times higher than the rest of Sweden, and this has been attributed to genetic selection for living in a remote, dispersed community. That interpretation is at odds with the high rates in Yugoslavia and Eire.

Dementia

It is possible that the dementias of later life occur with different frequencies in different areas of the world. In northern Europe and North America, the *overall* rates for dementias are very similar to each other and to those reported in Japan. An exception to this is the finding by Copeland *et al.* (1987), who have recently reported community prevalence rates for dementia in New York about twice those in London (5·7 and 10·1 per cent for men and women in New York, compared to 2·2 and 5·4 per cent respectively in London). This observation was based on the same case-finding instrument and the same diagnostic algorithm, AGECAT in both London and New York. Henderson (1986) reviewed 20 prevalence studies, examining rates for mild, moderate, and severe degrees of dementia and whether the sample had included persons living in institutions. The latter would obviously make a considerable difference to the estimates. Rates showed very great variation, almost certainly attributable to different case-finding criteria and methods. Jorm *et al.* (1987) compared prevalence estimates for senile dementia of Alzheimer type (SDAT) and multi-infarct (MID) or vascular dementia in five different world regions. In marked contrast to the pattern in the United Kingdom and some of the Scandinavian countries, the Japanese and Soviet studies showed a significant excess of MID and lower rates for SDAT. The Finnish and US studies revealed no significant differences, while the other Western countries showed an excess of AD over MID cases. An overview of these findings is shown in Table 3.3.

There are reports of an anecdotal type that SDAT is uncommon in Africa. Osuntokun (personal communication) found no cases of dementia among the elderly in a survey of 20 000 people in Nigeria, 5 per cent of whom were over 65 years old, although Lambo (1966) reported a substantial number of cases, both of senile and cerebrovascular dementia, in his Yoruba study. Even if one or both of the principal dementias were confirmed as being rare in less developed countries, this could be due to selective mortality: persons developing or likely to develop a dementia may die before the disorder becomes recognized. Furthermore, the elderly in such settings are themselves a survival élite who may be less vulnerable to dementia of either type. Even the correct determination of age is difficult when dates of birth are not recorded and birthdays are not celebrated. Nevertheless, it is still conceivable that the elderly in some non-industrialized countries develop a dementia of either type at much lower rates. Whereas this could be genetic in origin, some aspect of the diet or lifestyle may protect against dementia; or the unknown factors which cause SDAT may be absent from the environment. A low incidence of MID is more easily interpreted because of the relative rarity of cardiovascular disease.

Table 3.3 Relative prevalence of SDAT and MID.

Study	Age range	SDAT	MID
Japan			
Hasegawa (1979)	65+	1·2	2·7
Hasegawa *et al.* (1984)	65+	1·2	2·0
Kaneko (1975)	65+	1·9	5·5
Kaneko (1975)	60+	2·0	2·3
Karasawa *et al.* (1982)	65+	0·6	1·7
Russia			
Gavrilova (1984)	60+	1·4	2·0
Sternberg *et al.* (1978)	60+	2·8	3·5
Finland			
Mölsä *et al.* (1982)	65+	1·0	0·8
Sulkava *et al.* (1985)	65+	3·6	2·7
Scandinavia, other			
Åkesson (1969)	65+	1·0	0·3
Bollerup (1975)	70	1·3	1·9
UK			
Broe *et al.* (1976)	65+	5·4	1·9
Copeland (1981)	65+	2·0	0·3
Kay *et al.* (1964)	65+	4·4	4·0
Primrose (1962)	65+	2·7	0·9
USA			
Gurland *et al.* (1983)	65+	3·8	0·7
Folstein *et al.* (1985)	65+	2·0	2·8
Schoenberg *et al.* (1981)	60+	1·0	0·7

Prepared by Ailsa Korten.

Alcohol abuse

The great variation in the prevalence of alcoholism makes it clear that availability is only one factor in the causal chain. Where alcohol is not available, as in Muslim countries, there is virtually no morbidity. But within countries where it is consumed, there is considerable variation in the prevalence of alcohol-related problems. Indeed, there are important differences even within regions of a single country. These may provide clues to risk factors which in theory could be applied to primary prevention. Indices which may be compared are production rates, per capita consumption, deaths from cirrhosis, admission rates for treatment, alcohol-related offences, and prevalence estimates from population surveys. A comparison of different countries' alcohol production has been conducted by Walsh and Grant (1985).

Within single countries, there are now some carefully obtained estimates of prevalence in different regions. In the Epidemiologic Catchment Area studies, the lifetime prevalence of alcohol abuse or dependence was 15·7 per cent in St. Louis, 13·7 per cent in Baltimore, and 11·5 per cent in New Haven (Robins *et al.* 1984). These differences are not striking. In Britain, there has been a longstanding belief that alcoholism was more common in Scotland than England. Certainly, treatment rates suggested this, with as much as a 10-fold difference being cited. But recent evidence indicates that these figures do not reflect the true pattern. Latcham and Kreitman (1984) found that treatment rates for both men and women were virtually identical in the Scottish Highlands, Tayside, and Kent. Crawford *et al.* (1984, 1985) carried out population surveys of alcohol-related problems in these same areas. They found that there were minor differences in the proportion of abstainers and in mean levels of self-reported consumption, but these did not reflect the marked differences in official records for alcohol dependence. These workers concluded that there was little validity to the view that, at present, Scotland has higher levels either of consumption or of alcohol-related morbidity.

Suicide and parasuicide

Suicide There are striking differences within and between countries in their suicide rates. In interpreting this, many workers have rightly given close attention to the possibility that such differences are due to artefacts in recording and reporting of death by suicide (e.g. Barraclough 1969 and Sainsbury 1986). Although such artefacts undoubtedly play some part, there are almost certainly real differences between geographical areas and between countries. It was the evidence for differences between London boroughs which prompted Sainsbury (1955) to show the association between suicide rates and indices of social isolation. He first showed that the suicide rates of the 28 London boroughs were related to 17 indices of their social characteristics postulated as predisposing to suicide. For example, social isolation was measured indirectly by assessing the proportion of the borough population who lived alone or who were immigrants (in London as it was then). Both variables were associated with the borough's suicide rates. Sainsbury then examined the coroners' records for over 400 cases of suicide, finding that a higher proportion did indeed live alone or were immigrants, compared to the rest of the population.

More recently, attention has been given to the divergence of the English suicide rate from that of most other European nations. The suicide rate has shown a striking decrease in England, but everywhere else in Europe, except Greece, the rate has risen. The report of the World Health Organization (1982*a*) notes some of the possible explanations: an artefact in the data; the reduced availability of lethal poisons; better health and social services; and socioeconomic changes. An explanation based on artefact or inaccuracies in the reporting of suicide was ruled out. The decline in the English rate coincided closely with the reduction of carbon monoxide in domestic gas, but this is thought not to be a major reason for the change. Barraclough (1973), Barraclough and Hughes (1987), and Sainsbury *et al.* (1978) found that suicide rates had fallen not only in English towns changing to low levels of carbon monoxide, but also in towns where the level had remained lethal. Expansion of the telephone Samaritan service also coincided with the drop in England. But extensive investigation (Bagley 1968; Jennings *et al.* 1987) has shown that, although such services do much to help persons in distress, the evidence that they reduce suicide rates is at best equivocal. Because the clientele of the Samaritans is more like the parasuicide than the suicide population (Chowdhury & Kreitman 1971), it might be expected that it is the parasuicide rate which would drop, but this has not been found.

Sainsbury (1986) has provided a concise exposition of the social explanation for the changes in the pattern of suicide in Europe. Social events do affect national rates. He examined 15 social variables from 18 countries for the years 1961–63 and 1972–74. Some variables were presumed indicators of anomie (Durkheim 1897), of socioeconomic status, or of social change such as the status of women, or the alienation of the young and the elderly. In this elegant study, it was shown that suicide rose concurrently with increasing anomie and increasing affluence (as measured by rates of television ownership). Suicide in both sexes increased with the number of employed women. Unemployment, or more precisely the loss of employment and a change to relative poverty, was also shown to be associated with increased rates. The investigators then took five social variables as the best predictors of suicide: the divorce rate in each country, unemployment, homicide, women in employment, and the percentage of the population over the age of 15. They used these in a regression equation to predict the suicide rate of 18 European countries, then compared each of these rates with the observed rate. The finding is striking (Sainsbury 1986, p. 33): England and Greece showed a decrease, whereas the remaining European countries had increased rates, particularly Poland, The Netherlands, Denmark, Ireland, and Hungary. Social conditions, therefore, make a demonstrable and substantial contribution to the incidence of suicide.

Parasuicide Parasuicide rates vary between regions and are known to be markedly influenced by social variables. While acts of self-poisoning or self-injury are at present common amongst the urban young in many developed countries, particularly amongst the less favoured socioeconomic groups, such behaviour is reported to be exceptional in most developing countries. Parasuicide is associated with social disorganization, as evidenced by the ecological findings of Philip and McCulloch (1966) and Buglass *et al.* (1970). These workers found high rates for parasuicide in areas of Edinburgh characterized by high rates for juvenile delinquency, housing evictions, rent arrears, road accidents, cruelty to children, venereal disease, and illegitimate births. Cultural attitudes in such areas may increase the likelihood of parasuicide.

An important point in the epidemiology of parasuicide is that all of the above research was based on hospital data. Kennedy and Kreitman (1973) showed that a further 20–30 per cent of cases are known to general practitioners but not referred to a poisoning treatment centre or casualty department. There is no information on the further number of parasuicidal acts which do not reach primary health care, but it is highly improbable that these would appreciably alter the pattern described above.

SECULAR CHANGE

The incidence of some psychiatric disorders may change over time. The term secular comes from the Latin *saeculum* meaning an age or generation. This is of much intrinsic interest, because it stimulates speculation on the possible causes for the change. Often, however, the evidence for a real increase or decrease over time is difficult to establish. The social visibility of a disorder, or the proportion reaching professional attention, may account for an apparent change in incidence when the true base-rate in the population may not have altered. This may be the situation with schizophrenia, as discussed below. Next, even where a change in incidence is virtually certain, as with the contemporary increase in anorexia nervosa, the possible factors contributing to it are invariably multiple, and are confounded with others. This may make it very difficult to discern which amongst them may have an aetiological role. In short, this is an area which carries much popular appeal, but there are many technical difficulties in obtaining sound evidence.

Affective disorders

We have already discussed the changing pattern of suicide. Depressive disorders may have increased in incidence since the middle of the 20th century. The evidence for this is becoming impressive. Hagnell and his colleagues in Lund, Sweden, have been measuring the incidence of all psychiatric disorders, including depression, since the original survey of a total population by Essen-Möller (1956). They have now reported a marked increase in depressive disorders between 1947 and 1972 (Hagnell *et al.* 1982). This has taken place for both sexes, as Fig. 3.1 reproduced from their data shows. There was a small drop in the incidence of severe depressions, possibly due to the advent of effective drugs, but the rate for mild and moderate depression increased markedly. For young men aged 20–39 years, the incidence rose 10-fold between the 1947–57 and 1957–72 periods.

In the course of the Epidemiologic Catchment Area studies, it was found that the lifetime prevalence reported by each age group was actually *lower* for major depression in those aged 65 and over than in younger adults. Yet these older persons had had the longest period at risk. A similar trend was also present for dysthymia, though it was less marked. This finding deserves cautious interpretation because it could easily be an artefact of self-reporting, whereby older people fail to recall earlier episodes. But it could also be due to a true historical increase in incidence affecting younger persons, consistent with the Lundby findings.

Klerman *et al.* (1985) examined 2289 first degree relatives of 523 probands with affected disorder, using the Schedule for Affective

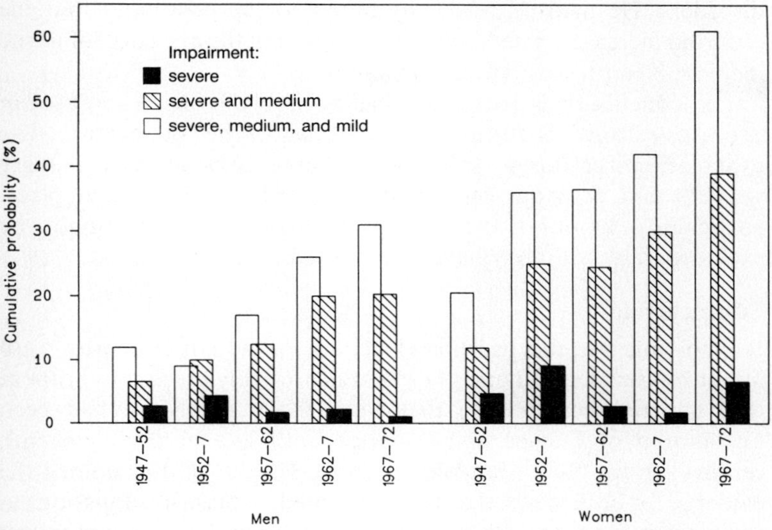

Fig. 3.1 The cumulative probability of contracting depression before the age of 80, with the 25-year span divided into 5-year periods. (From Hagnell *et al.*, 1982. *Psychological Medicine*, **12,** 279–89, Cambridge University Press. Reproduced with kind permission of the authors and publisher.)

Disorders and Schizophrenia (SADS). They found that rates for having had an episode of major depression at some time up to the interview were higher in successively younger birth cohorts. Klerman and his colleagues considered alternative interpretations, including memory effects in reporting, selective mortality, or a greater readiness recently to acknowledge having depressive symptoms. They hypothesized that the observed increase is due to the emergence of a significant discrepancy between expectations of future personal and economic rewards and the perceived opportunities for the attainment of these rewards.

Another hypothesis is that the increase has biological causes, such as viral or other infections, changes in dietary practices, or the ingestion of environmental pollutants. A full account of the US evidence and its interpretation is set out in Klerman (1987). In Mannheim, Germany, Häfner (1985) examined in some detail the evidence for an increase in both depression and other psychiatric disorders. He paid particular attention to the possibility that the reported increase is artefactual, but found that the evidence for a true increase is impressive, though incomplete.

The conclusion is that there has probably been an increase in depressive disorders during the second half of the 20th century. The explanation for this is unknown. Whereas psychosocial changes which could promote depression have indisputably taken place, particularly amongst the young, biological factors cannot be excluded, and both may have contributed.

Schizophrenia

It is possible that this psychosis was rare, or did not even exist, until about 200 years ago. Torrey (1980) was probably the first to propose that schizophrenia, unlike manic-depressive psychosis, had been uncommon in Europe and America until late in the eighteenth century. In his 1982 Maudsley Lecture, Hare (1983) examined the evidence for both views: that the undoubted increase in admissions to asylums in the late 18th century was due wholly to nosocomical factors, whereby the incidence of schizophrenia was really constant, but more cases reached hospital; or that there was indeed an increase in incidence.

Torrey (1980) proposed that schizophrenia is curiously absent from the descriptions of mental disorder in classical Greece or Rome. But Jeste *et al.* (1985) have argued that this may be due to the disorder's lower social salience and the lack of adequate terminology to describe it. They found some earlier accounts from India in the first century AD and Britain in the Middle Ages which might be descriptions of schizophrenia. Torrey (1980) also suggested that schizophrenia may have been absent or rare in other parts of the world, prior to European contact. Both Torrey and Hare point to the well-documented change in the clinical manifestations of schizophrenia during the 20th century. The disorder has diminished in severity (Ødegard 1967) and catatonia has become very much rarer.

A social hypothesis for an increase has been argued by J. Cooper and Sartorius (1977). They suggest that several factors associated with industrialization may have promoted the manifestation of schizophrenia, especially in its severe or chronic forms. These factors are: a change towards living in nuclear families in large communities; specialization of work and social roles, so that these become much tighter and less flexible in their demands; recognition of mental disorders as separate from physical illness; and the survival of more infants and children, some of whom may have increased vulnerability to schizophrenia. These proposals are entirely compatible with biological explanations.

The attraction of the 'slow epidemic' hypothesis is its utility, as Hare has pointed out. Unlike the contrary view, that schizophrenia has always been present, that its incidence has not greatly changed, and that it is and always has been ubiquitous, the slow epidemic hypothesis parsimoniously explains the following: the distinct possibility that its incidence did rise in the 18th century, leading to the fairly abrupt building of mental hospitals in the Western world; the inadequacy of an exclusively genetic aetiology; the findings on seasonality of birth; the relatively better prognosis for schizophrenia in developing countries (WHO 1979; Sartorius *et al.* 1987); and recent evidence on changes in brain function and ventricular size (Murray *et al.* 1985). Finally, and most powerful of all, the hypothesis carries optimism for treatment, and heuristic value by providing direction for research (Hare 1983).

Dementia

The prevalence of dementia for total populations or countries, expressed as the number of cases per 1000 adults, has indisputably increased during the twentieth century. But this is wholly attributable to a considerable expansion in the elderly population at risk, particularly the very elderly. This demographic shift has been very thoroughly documented for all World Regions in three World Health Organization publications (WHO 1982*a*, *b*, 1984), which are excellent reference sources.

It is nevertheless possible that, alongside this, a decrease in incidence may have taken place within the last two or three decades. Hagnell (1966, 1981) has been determining the incidence of mental disorders in a total population in Sweden since it was first examined by Essen-Möller in 1947. In this unique work, Hagnell *et al.* (1981) were able to compare the incidence of dementia in the elderly over two time-periods. They reported that the incidence had dropped appreciably. This drop was later shown to hold both for SDAT and MID (Hagnell *et al.* 1983). In a subsequent paper, they re-analysed their data including those who had moved into Lundby in the 1947–57 period. No statistically significant change in either incidence or prevalence could then be detected (Rorsman *et al.* 1986). Because of the chronicity of dementia, a detectable drop in incidence, even if it were present, is unlikely to alter the total prevalence to any appreciable extent, so that it would be false to expect any decrease in the burden on services.

MACROSOCIAL FACTORS

On a few occasions, social scientists have proposed some property of a society as a significant causal factor for mental disorders. The implication has been that there are social forces at work additional to those which operate in interpersonal relationships; that is, they operate at a societal rather than an individual level. These are macrosocial and have their origin in constructs such as the overall pattern of living, what is valued by people as important, the strength of beliefs, and the extent to which individuals experience themselves as part of a larger social organism. A recurrent notion has been that weakening of such cohesive forces promotes mental disorder. Durkheim (1897) drew attention to the link he believed existed between suicide in Europe and the state of 'anomie'. By the latter, he meant a breakdown of the collective conscience, with a resulting deficiency in behavioural norms. He believed that certain social forces bind together the members of a society and that individuals are adversely affected where this is weakened.

More recently, D. C. Leighton *et al.* (1963*a*) described 'sociocultural disintegration' as a condition which develops in a community and which is associated, they proposed, with increased psychiatric morbidity. This condition was thought to be characterized by a predominance of 'centrifugal forces' which impaired the society's capacity for adaptation. It has been difficult to obtain a clear definition of the concept, but at least 10 components have been proposed for those sociocultural conditions which may be related to psychiatric disorder (the diagnoses not being specified): those conditions which interfere with sentiments of physical security, securing sexual satisfaction, expression of hostility, giving and receiving love, obtaining recognition, expressing spontaneity, feeling oriented in terms of place in society and the place of others, membership in a well-defined human group, belonging to a moral order, and being right in what one does (D. C. Leighton *et al.* 1963*a*, p. 366, *et seq.*). Such constructs do not readily lend themselves to epidemiological investigation. In terms of epidemiological method, it has not proved easy to measure sociocultural disintegration as the independent variable, free of the manifestations of psychiatric disorders themselves. Furthermore, the cross-sectional designs which have been used are very limited in establishing causal effects. The only design which could show that such disintegration generates an increased incidence would be a prospective longitudinal study of a community as it underwent disintegration. A scientifically satisfactory study based on such a natural experiment is unlikely to be practicable.

In the Stirling County and Yoruba studies, the Leightons and their colleagues were examining a rich pastiche of adverse social conditions (A. H. Leighton *et al.* 1963; D. C. Leighton *et al.* 1963*a*, *b*). They believed that these combined to make a conceptual entity and that this was pathogenic. The morbidity generated was thought to be non-specific, so that no particular mental disorder was implicated. But it is highly improbable that a pathogenic effect, if it exists, would hold across the various major categories of psychiatric disorder. Most difficult of all, however, there was a serious likelihood in the above surveys that the independent and dependent variables were confounded. That is, there were social functioning items presented as part of the symptom inventory, and some of the social functioning measures referred to symptoms of mental disorder.

TRANSCULTURAL STUDIES AND OTHER MACROSOCIAL FACTORS

In trying to delineate macrosocial factors which may influence mental health, much interesting material has been accumulated in the field of transcultural psychiatry. Readers are referred to key sources for this subject, such as Yap (1974), Kiev (1972), Murphy (1982), Leff (1981), Marsella *et al.* (1979), and Cox (1986). Transcultural psychiatry examines patterns of morbidity across different cultures, and attempts to interpret observed differences in terms of these cultures. This paradigm holds for aetiology and course, but also for patterns of help-seeking and treatment. Macrosocial factors have consistently been invoked to account for apparently high rates of some disorders, or the apparent paucity of others.

Murphy (1982) has rightly advocated caution in comparing hospitalization rates, because these are influenced by many factors other than the true incidence in a community. He concluded that some national groups probably do have higher morbidity. One example he gives is the southwest Croatians, who seem unduly vulnerable to psychopathology in general, carrying higher rates in a community prevalence survey for affective disorder and other psychoses besides schizophrenia (see this chapter, p. 53), but also higher hospitalization rates for coronary heart disease, hypertension, asthma, and cerebral thrombosis. The reasons for this, whether they be macrosocial, genetic, or environmental, have not yet been determined. Murphy gives as a second example the Singapore Indians, whom he describes as having high rates for suicide, schizophrenia, other psychoses, hypertension, adult asthma, and juvenile delinquency. But as other Indian populations overseas, as in Fiji, Mauritius, and Trinidad, do not appear also to have increased morbidity, Murphy thought the difference could be due to the Singaporean Indians' having minority status. The Hutterites in the United States were at first thought to have a high level of mental health, presumably attributable to their well-ordered life-style and religious practice. Whereas this is true for antisocial behaviour and personality disorder, it is now clear that the Hutterites are not protected from affective disorder.

Brewin (1980) pursued the lead that Asian immigrants in Britain seemed to have low rates for psychiatric treatment. This might have been due to some macrosocial protective factor, to their being psychologically more resistant, or to their using other sources of help for psychiatric disorders. He showed that Asian and English people consulted general practitioners at the same rate, but that Asians with psychiatric symptoms were less likely to be recognized as unwell, or referred to psychiatric services. The original observation had no relationship to macrosocial factors.

Transcultural psychiatry clearly has a major investment in the potential explanatory power of macrosocial and cultural factors. Most of us feel intuitively that they are very likely to be important determinants of mental health throughout the life-cycle. Recurrently, however, major difficulties emerge in finding the evidence. It is very difficult to measure morbidity in the same way in two contrasted cultures; and it is equally difficult to measure macrosocial factors. Even if they are so apparent that they may not need to be quantified, there is then the problem that some other social factors may co-exist with them, and be equally powerful but unobserved. Furthermore, the biological and genetic conditions are obviously going to be different, so that a purely macrosocial explanation becomes impossible.

For future studies of macrosocial determinants of mental disorders, the best that is likely to be achieved is to repeat a population survey *in the same community* after some marked change has taken place, probably a decade or more later. The same case-finding methods would need to be used, and the assumption made that the composition of the population had not changed in the interval. A useful yield of knowledge seems unlikely in this matter, considering the effort required and the methodological issues to be confronted.

War

There is evidence that admission rates to mental hospitals decreased during World War II. This observation has been extended to imply that war causes a decrease in psychiatric morbidity, but the evidence for such a view is quite inadequate. Rates for treated morbidity cannot be taken as a valid index of total morbidity: access to services are obviously likely to be reduced in wartime. Exposure to military action is itself associated with considerable morbidity, so that rates might be expected to rise, both in military personnel and their families. The theory to support a decrease in morbidity is a simple one: during wartime, individuals share an externalization of stresses in living, where these are seen to arise principally from a common enemy. Some social forces bind communities together in the face of this. Material hardship is somehow not seen by individuals as a stressor, nor does the loss of life cause increased morbidity in the bereaved, although these losses are usually numerous. The conclusion must be that the hypothesis is a doubtful one; and that there are at present insufficient data to uphold it. Nor is it likely to be easily settled. That would require a community survey of a large sample, including all its menfolk, before and during a major war. Such data are unlikely to be obtained.

Rapid modernization

The notion has long been held that the pressures of urban living in industrialized societies have caused an increase in mental disorders. Some distinguished writers have looked carefully at this argument and the evidence they could find to support or refute it. At La Salpêtrière in Paris, Esquirol (1967) and in Germany, Aschaffenburg (1915) were principal contributors, as Lewis (1967) described in his essay 'Ebb and flow in social psychiatry'. But these authors had only mental hospital admission rates as their measure of morbidity over time. Likewise, the celebrated study of Goldhamer and Marshall (1953) entitled *Psychosis and civilization*, was based only on admission rates to Massachusetts mental hospitals. Such data may indeed reflect morbidity as it is really occurring, but they are also strongly influenced by the utilization of services by the public. Even if incidence or prevalence rates at the community level were available, the argument for the pathogenicity of modernization is often ill-balanced and selective.

In its contemporary form it holds that, as less developed countries undergo transition to an industrialized economy, a number of far-reaching changes commonly accompany this; and that further changes in living patterns are brought about by the new technologies. A well-known exposition of this can be found in Toffler (1971, 1980). Major alterations have come about in patterns of work, of family life, and traditional beliefs and values. Technical advances take place in communication and in the transport of persons and consumer goods. Large numbers may quite abruptly be exposed to mass communication, including television, which often portrays a standard of living and behavioural pattern previously unknown to them. They may be exposed to foreign visitors and tourists in large numbers. There is a tendency for rural–urban migration, particularly of the young. Traditional family patterns and religious practices may be shed. Marked differences in values and attributes may emerge between two, three, or even four generations, often living in one household. Dietary habits and the use of leisure are likely to alter substantially. These processes are called modernization or rapid social change. They are believed to be stressful and to be of legitimate concern for public health, particularly in the area of psychiatric illness, including alcohol and drug dependency. But it seems equally reasonable to argue that modernization may bring a number of benefits: people often have better physical health, a lower infant mortality rate, increased life expectancy, better housing and sanitation, and improved opportunities for work, leisure, and family life. Such changes, together with the indisputable adaptability of most people, make it just as likely that modernization is not the threat to mental health which is commonly inferred.

Clearly there are shared components in urbanization, regional variation, secular change, and modernization. These components take the form of social phenomena and alterations in life-style affecting large segments of a population. Their influence on mental health is often highly plausible, but it has proved difficult to dissect them into clearly defined entities and to investigate their independent effects.

4

Life experiences as causes of mental disorders: the main hypotheses

Childhood separation and contextual effects; parental style and its implications for clinical practice and prevention; adverse life-events; extreme experiences; bereavement; unemployment; social support.

We listed in Table 3.1 (p. 31) those sociodemographic factors and experiences which have been proposed as related to mental disorders. Most of them have been systematically investigated in clinical and epidemiological studies. We now examine those which are truly social, in that they consist of exposures to or experiences with others. The topics selected for examination here are childhood separation, parental style, adverse life-events and extreme experiences, bereavement, expressed emotion, unemployment, and social support.

CHILDHOOD SEPARATION

The work of Bowlby (1969, 1973, 1980) ranks amongst the most significant this century in the theory of human social development and mental health. It has established the nature of the tie between mothers and children, emphasizing its phylogenetic origins in higher primates and its importance for species survival in a primeval environment. Bowlby's theory of attachment has promoted the acquisition of knowledge in two areas: how infants and children behave when separated from their mother; and, of much more clinical relevance, how the relationship with parents may contribute to psychopathology later in life. The general hypothesis has been that separation or threatened separation from the mother leads not only to distress in the child at the time, but causes intrapsychic changes which predispose to depression or, in some instances, abnormal personality in adulthood. A succinct overview of the theory, its origins, predictions, and application to psychotherapy has been set out by Bowlby in his Fiftieth Maudsley Lecture (Bowlby 1977*a*).

We have emphasized earlier how necessary it is to specify the independent or predictor variables. Attachment theorists have taken pains to do this. Bowlby (1977*a*, p. 206) gives a useful list of pathogenic behaviours in parents. They are:

(1) one or both parents being persistently unresponsive to a child's care-eliciting behaviour, or being actively disparaging and rejecting;
(2) discontinuities of parenting, occurring more or less frequently, including periods in hospital or institution;
(3) persistent threats by parents not to love a child, used as a means of controlling him;
(4) threats by parents to abandon the family, used either as a method of disciplining the child or as a way of coercing a spouse;
(5) threats by one parent either to desert or even to kill the other, or else to commit suicide (each of these being more common than might be supposed);
(6) inducing a child to feel guilty by claiming that his behaviour is or will be responsible for the parent's illness or death.

These behaviours may induce a state of 'anxious attachment' in which the child, or indeed an adolescent or adult, is in a more-or-less constant state of apprehension, lest he or she should lose the one person who is of most emotional significance. But there is a further issue which has to be specified. This is the social and affective context in which separations or permanent loss take place; and the quality of subsequent parenting available to the child from others. Rutter (1972) has justifiably given emphasis to this in his review of the effects of maternal deprivation.

No one doubts that separation from the mother causes distress in the young; and that it is fairly consistently followed by a sequence of behaviours and affective states, characterized as protest, despair and, if the separation continues, emotional detachment. These patterns seem to hold in other higher primates: they are phylogenetically established, probably being hard-wired into the brain. But for longer-term consequences, the evidence is much less persuasive. Under the stimulus of attachment theory, many studies have been conducted which compare the reported separation experiences of adults who have had a particular psychiatric disorder with some unafflicted group. Both case-control designs on treated samples as well as community surveys have been used (Birtchnell 1970, 1980). The results have been inconsistent and confusing. Some studies have found an increased frequency of separation or loss of either parent in persons with adult psychiatric disorders; other studies have failed to find a difference. The issues at stake in this matter are so fundamental for progress in social psychiatry that we shall now look at them closely; the principles involved have wider applicability. It seems that the following has taken place:

1. Based on naturalistic observation, a proposition has been made about the effect of separating children from their parents, particularly their mothers, and the damage this may do to their mental health in later years.

2. This hypothesis was derived in part by clinicians working with disordered persons. They were not in a position to pay equal attention to those who had had childhood loss or separation but *did not subsequently become disordered, or did not reach professional attention.*

3. The general hypothesis was avidly received, both by the professions caring for children and the research community. Both were receptive to such an idea: the professions because it provided a rational basis for policy, and for greater humanity towards children likely to be deprived of maternal care; the research community because there had been a dearth of ideas to explain the genesis of mental disorders in experiential terms.

4. The hypothesis then developed many variants. The dependent variable has been depression, schizophrenia, parasuicide, various neurotic disorders, and an undifferentiated clinical series of psychiatric symptoms or personality disorders, including antisocial or criminal behaviour. The predictor variable has also varied between mother–child separations of some weeks to permanent loss, including death of the mother. Separations from the father have likewise been explored, although much less intensively.

5. The data to test these hypotheses have often been based on a case-control design: that is, a sample of persons in contact with services, usually adults, has been contrasted with some comparison group by obtaining a history of deprivation or separation retrospectively, usually from the respondents themselves. The cases have often been symptomatic, or at least in some personal difficulty, at the time of the interview, rather than being persons who had recovered from a

past episode. The possibility of information bias due to 'effort after meaning' must be appreciable (see p. 84), whereby those with psychiatric symptoms make greater efforts than those without to recall adverse experiences in the past to account for their present state. There is also the possibility of an association between parental loss in childhood and help-seeking in adult life (Fig. 4.1). That is, those who reach services may be more likely to have had parental loss in childhood. Other studies have been based on community samples, where the help-seeking factor can be discounted, but where the severity of disorders tends to be less.

6. The possibility of confounding by related variables has tended to be ignored. Such variables could be demographic or constitutional. How they may act as confounders is shown in Fig. 4.1. For example, if the cases differ from the controls in social class during childhood, or in the size of the family and their position in it, the likelihood of experiencing separations will also be different. Again, a genetic predisposition to a psychiatric disorder, including abnormal personality, may be associated with an increased probability of breakdown of marriage or suicide in either parent. Demographic or constitutional factors may also influence the likelihood of reaching professional services.

7. Finally, most studies have looked for a simple association between parental loss and adult mental disorder. They have not considered more developed aetiological models where several vari-

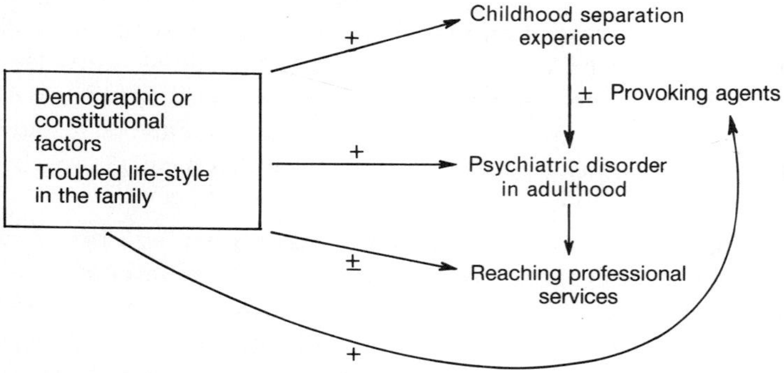

Fig. 4.1 Childhood separation and adult psychiatric disorder: a possible model.

ables co-act, some as vulnerability factors and others as precipitating agents, as proposed by Brown and Harris (1978) and Harris *et al.* (1986). As Birtchnell (1980) has emphasized, simple one-to-one causal relationships are improbable in human development.

Conclusion

For the present, it is probably best to accept the conclusion of Tennant *et al.* (1980) regarding the specific case of parental death and adult depression. Although they focused deliberately on this association rather than on less specified associations, they were led to two opposing conclusions: that a causal effect exists but is highly specific, working only in certain sociodemographic groups, so that there is frequently a failure to establish an association; or that there is an ubiquitous effect, but that it is weak. There is some recent evidence to support the first of these. Surtees (1984) found in the Edinburgh Survey that early maternal loss was powerfully associated with high case-rates for non-psychotic disorder, but only in women who were separated or divorced. Harris *et al.* (1986) has drawn attention to this need to consider grouping of variables, in which a causal effect may emerge only in interaction with other factors.

Birtchnell (1970, 1980) has investigated parental loss for nearly two decades, finding a positive association in his earlier studies, but none in later ones. He concludes that the actual death of a parent is undoubtedly disturbing but does not cause lasting harm, and that any ill effects which do follow are related to inadequate mothering subsequent to the loss. That is, the crucial variable is the quality of later care given to the child. This conclusion is also reached by Harris *et al.* (1986) from their Walthamstow study. In their Islington study, Brown and his colleagues found a link between poor parental care in childhood and low self-esteem in adulthood (Brown and Harris 1986; Brown *et al.* 1986*a*). The evidence thus points consistently to the pathogenicity not of parental loss *per se*, but to the behaviour of parents or parent surrogates during childhood. In this way, research on the behaviour of parents is a logical sequel to earlier work on the categorical variable of separation or loss.

PARENTAL STYLE

This is a recent arrival in the list of postulated experiential factors. It refers to the pattern of childrearing to which people have been exposed. The hypothesis is that the experience of high levels of controlling behaviour, but low levels of care and concern by parents, confers increased risk of developing neurotic disorders in adulthood, particularly depression. It is proposed that this effect is mediated through decrements in parental care jeopardizing self-esteem, and through parental control having adverse effects on the development of social competence. This hypothesis has arisen from two complementary sources. Attachment theory as developed by Bowlby construes healthy parents as providing a secure base and encouraging exploration from it. Pathogenic parents, by contrast, are uncaring, unresponsive, and rejecting. Furthermore, instead of encouraging gradual separation and independence, they may be excessively controlling, often in a manner which ensures that the young person does not have opportunities to venture away from them.

The second source of the hypothesis is from psychometric studies of the behaviour and attitudes of parents. With remarkable consistency, a number of factor analytic studies have pointed to the existence of two principal variables: the first is behaviour characterized by care, concern, and affection; the second is emphasis by a parent on control and a tendency towards overprotection. The consistency of these findings is impressive (Roe and Siegelman 1963; Schaefer 1965; Raskin *et al.* 1971). Parker (1983*a*) has drawn the evidence together, providing a critical review of this literature and what it suggests.

Instruments

The appeal of the hypothesis has stimulated the development of instruments to measure the two dimensions of care and control. The Parental Bonding Instrument (PBI) was developed by Parker (1983*a*) in Sydney and Oxford, while the EMBU (Swedish acronym for 'own memories of childhood rearing experiences') was developed by Perris *et al.* (1980) in Umeå. Both instruments were prompted by an appreciation of the need to explore potentially important interpersonal experiences in childhood. Both depend on self-reported information about past behaviour and attitudes on the part of the respondent's parents.

Extensive developmental work has gone into assessing the reliability and validity of the PBI. Validity is a critical issue here, as we are seeking information about interactions often far in the past, lasting over 10 to 15 years, and we are doing so by self-report. The validity of the PBI has been examined in a number of ways: comparing the reports of siblings on their parents; having pairs of siblings complete the PBI for themselves, and as though they were the other sibling; and comparing the scores of subjects with the self-report of the mothers themselves, as they believed they had behaved. In all of these, very satisfactory validity has been found.

Reliability has been shown to be very high. Indeed, it was high even when scores for depressed patients were compared with those obtained nine weeks later, after symptoms had diminished. Here the correlations were between +0·87 to 0·92. This is an important observation, because depressed persons might be expected, while depressed, to report their parents in an unfavourable light. The possibility of such information bias deserves further careful checking before it can be fully excluded.

The inspiration of the EMBU and the hypotheses tested by its authors came from exploratory studies of how depressed patients recalled their parents' behaviour towards them (Raskin *et al.* 1971; Jacobson *et al.* 1975). Perris *et al.* (1980) were able to establish three factors from data on both normal and depressed subjects: rejection, emotional warmth, and overprotection. More recent work with the EMBU (Arrindell *et al.* 1986*a*, *b*) has resulted in a two-factor model, care and protection, suggesting striking similarities to the PBI research.

The evidence

The nature of the hypothesis lends itself to case-control studies, because it refers to a past exposure on which information necessarily has to be obtained retrospectively, usually by self-report. The studies done so far have, not surprisingly, been mainly cross-sectional, comparing cases of designated disorders with a comparison group of mentally healthy persons. Both the work of Parker (1983*a*, 1983*b*, 1984, 1988); Parker *et al.* 1987) and Perris *et al.* (1986) have shown that neurotic disorders, particularly depression, have a strong association with 'affectionless control'. Parker found that both mothers and fathers were assigned to the low-care/high-protection quadrant by patients with depressive neurosis, social phobias, anxiety-neurosis, and agoraphobia. A weaker association was found in schizophrenia.

Perris *et al.* (1986), using the EMBU, have obtained strikingly similar findings. Patients with depression, particularly unipolar, but also neurotic and unspecified depressive disorder, rated their parents lower than controls on emotional warmth and higher in overprotection. They concluded that an upbringing deprived of affection may be an important psychological risk factor in the background of depressive disorders. It is impressive that two independent groups, with different frames of reference and different instruments, have obtained similar findings.

Interpretation

This association calls for very careful interpretation because, if it were conclusively shown to be a causal one, the implications for childrearing and primary prevention would be profound. Parker (1983*a*, 1984, 1987) has set out the possible interpretations:

1. The PBI may not be a valid measure of actual parental behaviour, in that responses are significantly influenced by personality attributes, which lead both to high scores for neurotic symptoms and the perception of parental behaviour as unfavourable. The evidence from validity studies runs counter to this as a major explanation.

2. One or more confounding variables lead on the one hand to symptoms, or to reporting of them on research instruments; and on the other to reports of 'affectionless control' in parents. No such confounding variable has yet been found, though it may exist. Parker's studies were able to exclude social desirability, neuroticism and genetic factors. A link was demonstrated between depression in the offspring and parental anomalies, as scored by the mothers about themselves (Parker 1983*a*). This is evidence against reports of parental behaviour being contaminated by mood.

3. The association may be valid, but the direction of causality may be, in a sense, reversed: affectionless control may be elicited in parents by children who will later develop neurotic disorders and depression.

4. Affectionless control may indeed have a causal influence on the subsequent development of neurosis. One way this might be mediated is through the induction of anxious attachment as described in attachment theory (Bowlby 1977*a*).

To these interpretations, a further one may be added: in the studies based on clinical samples, there may be ascertainment bias, whereby these are not fully representative of all cases of the neurotic disorders.

The association may have more to do with having sought professional help than with the genesis of the symptoms themselves. That is, affectionless control may be associated with help-seeking, not psychiatric morbidity itself. A similar proposition has been made for life-events (Andrews and Tennant 1978*a*) and social support (Henderson *et al.* 1978*a*).

Conclusions

Parker (1984) has concluded that affectionless control may be

> irrelevant to the onset of certain psychiatric disorders (e.g. manic-depressive psychosis), be an antecedent to, and a possible causal influence on other psychiatric disorders (e.g. neurosis), be a consequence of chronic disorder in a child (e.g. asthma), and be a possible influence on the course of certain psychiatric disorders (e.g. schizophrenia).

Confirmation of the parental style hypothesis can now be obtained by only one design: a prospective study of the incidence of psychiatric disorders in two samples who differ only in their exposure to affectionless control during childhood. This would be a demanding but important undertaking, the results of which could have a powerful influence on strategies for the prevention in childhood of mental disorders in adult life. But it is very unlikely to be practicable. It is most unlikely that this could be achieved with true random allocation in an experimental design, for ethical reasons. This would leave the difference in parental style open to confounding by other factors.

Application to treatment and prevention

Meanwhile, psychiatry has the option of assuming that affectionless control *is* an undesirable style for bringing up children; that attempts to reverse its possible consequences are justified; and that efforts to discourage it might be a valuable exercise in the primary prevention of some mental disorders. The provision of genuine affection, together with opportunities for independent exploration of the environment without inappropriate constraint, is after all unlikely to be harmful. By contrast, there is now much in the evidence above to suggest that the opposite style of parental behaviour may induce vulnerability to neurotic illness in adult life. In this way, the parental style hypothesis carries one major asset: it provides a fairly clear prescription to parents about how to give their children a higher probability of having mental health in adulthood.

Readers may ask themselves if there may be some common ground between the constructs of affectionless control and high expressed emotion (see p. 148). For example, both imply some hostility towards the target individual; both carry the wish to alter his or her behaviour; and both imply that the parent or close relative may be intolerant and given to criticism of others. In this way, it is possible that the apparent overlap between the factors identified in the work on parental style and on expressed emotion may carry some clinical and theoretical significance. It points to a potentially rich research agenda on mental illness and family interaction. A distinction to note is that the parental style hypothesis is mainly concerned with aetiology, whereas expressed emotion is concerned with relapse.

ADVERSE LIFE-EVENTS

The notion that emotionally distressing experiences may be followed by physical or mental illness is an ancient one. Physicians in the classical era were well aware that misfortune often preceded the onset of illness, but unlike contemporary practitioners, they did not make a distinction between physical and mental disorders. The French physiologist Claude Bernard was the first to propose that the attempts of living organisms to adapt to their environment can be closely related to disease processes. Systematic enquiry into adverse experiences began under the impetus of work by Hinkle and Wolff (1957*a*). In their important paper, 'The nature of man's adaptation to his total environment and the relation of this to illness', they concluded from their longitudinal studies on three groups of people that 'clusters of illness most often appear when a person is having difficulty adapting to his environment as perceived by him'. They also noted that individuals differed in the amount of illness they had, and that this appeared to be due in part to '*inherent differences in their adaptive capacities*' (our italics), as well as different levels of difficulty encountered. In a parallel paper, Hinkle and Wolff (1957*b*) made the important suggestion for public health that, in the general population, those who are attempting to adapt to difficult life situations contribute substantially to the total burden of morbidity. That is, a group exists in any population who have an excess of both physical and mental disorders. Indeed, all of these ideas applied to both physical and mental illness. The emphasis on only psychiatric disorders emerged some time later.

A major advance in psychiatry and social medicine came with the development of the Social Readjustment Rating Scale, constructed by Holmes and Rahe (1967). The availability of this instrument kindled an interest in the role of recent stress in the onset of illness, a hypothesis which had hitherto lacked a method for its systematic study. Holmes and Rahe believed that the important attribute of life-events was the amount of adaptation required of the individual. Although subsequently modified by others, the original paradigm and prototype life-event inventory was the progenitor of a massive body of research. Much of it has been of mixed quality, but the experience gained has led to a clearer awareness of the technical difficulties in measuring adversity and in attempting to show its causal effects. We now examine some of these issues and how they have been tackled.

The development of methods

What the investigator usually seeks is a method for measuring the stress to which individuals have recently been exposed. Stress is defined as 'a condition of things compelling or characterized by strained effort' (*Shorter Oxford English Dictionary*). The events or circumstances responsible are stressors. Because of variability between individuals in their constitution and current environmental conditions, a particular stressor may not cause the same level of stress to each person. This variability of impact has been a major technical challenge. Stress cannot be measured directly by asking the individual, because the response would be open to confounding by his affective state at the time. This problem has therefore had to be resolved in some research designs by making the considerable assumption that a given experience, such as losing one's job has, on average, the same impact on all individuals. A very different approach, as we shall see, is the Bedford College method, which takes into account the personal and social context of the event, thereby achieving some expression of its impact on a particular individual in a particular context. Most research has focused on temporally discrete events, but many believe it is also important to include longstanding stressors, such as the chronic difficulties which Brown and Harris (1978) have included in their measures.

Typically, the period of exposure being considered has been the previous 12 months, although this is almost certainly too long a span of time. In weaker studies, the exact date of an event within the period is not ascertained. In better studies, efforts may be made to date the event within the period, placing it in time as accurately as possible, particularly in relation to the time of onset of symptoms. We can be confident that the event and the subsequent onset of a disorder are fairly close in time (Brown and Birley 1968): events long past are unlikely to have an enduring pathogenic effect unless they are exceptionally severe, such as concentration camp experiences. Surtees and Ingham (1980) have developed an attractive mathematical model for the decay of the impact of adversity over time (see also Surtees, 1988).

In conducting research into life-events, there are at least 10 demanding questions which have to be faced:

1. What is an event?
2. How are those events which are to be counted to be defined?
3. How is the actual occurrence of events to be elicited?
4. How are the events to be graded: on unpleasantness, the amount of change required, or some other dimension?
5. How can the measurement of events be made free of contamination by the illness itself, as sick people may report having recently had worse experiences?
6. Should the rest of the individual's life situation, which determines the context of the event, be taken into account?
7. Should the individual's constitutional vulnerability and his reaction to the event be considered?
8. Can a reverse direction of causality be excluded, whereby the illness itself, or its prodromata, cause the life-event?
9. Can confounding by a third set of variables be excluded, such as certain personality traits predisposing both to a psychiatric disorder and to the recruitment of events and difficulties? This raises the important distinction between 'dependent' and 'independent' events or difficulties, introduced by Brown and Harris (1978).
10. What is the strength of any demonstrable contribution made by life-events to the onset of a specific disorder?

On these 10 issues depends the value of the information obtained. Useful accounts of how to tackle them have been provided by Sarason and Spielberger (1979), Dohrenwend and Dohrenwend (1981), and Paykel (1983).

Two methods for collecting information are at present in use. In the inventory method developed by Holmes and Rahe (1967), a list of experiences is presented to the respondent, either on paper for self-completion or by reading them out. The respondent then endorses those items which most closely describe events or experiences in the specified period. The procedure typically takes 15 to 20 minutes. Each item carries a particular score. These are added to give a total score for the individual. A very different approach is the interview method developed by Brown and Harris (1978) at Bedford College. In this, the individual's experience of events and difficulties is first determined by interview, using a list of possible occurrences. Events which could be due to the disorder or its prodromata are later excluded, so that only 'independent' events are considered. The context of each event is determined by obtaining detailed information on the individual's life situation at the time, including his or her preparedness and the personal implications of the experience. This procedure may take two to three hours. The information is then presented to a group of trained raters. According to a documented procedure which includes definitions, guide-notes and examples, these raters then decide whether the event or difficulty was marked, moderate or mild. A severe event is one which is rated both as being marked and having a score of 2 on its 'subject focus', meaning that the event is likely to have had a substantial impact on the respondent, if not also on others. Deliberately, they do not take into account the individual's subjective or personal response to the experience, or his assessment of the severity of the event. Precautions are also taken to keep the raters unaware if the person has symptoms or not. In these ways, the Bedford College method differs fundamentally from the checklist approach, both in how exposure to events are elicited and how each is rated for severity. It also requires training and the allocation of much more time.

What is to be counted?

The issue here is the universe of experiences which the investigator wishes to cover. What is to be counted may be selected by the respondent from within a predetermined list, such as the 43 set out in the original inventory by Holmes and Rahe (1967), or the headings in the Brown and Harris interview. Clearly, a list may be more appropriate for one population than another, by reason of culture or demographic characteristics. A further issue is the temporal characteristics of the experience, whether it is quite discrete, such as a burglary; or something likely to have prolonged significance, such as having a bereavement; or whether it is not an event but a longstanding difficulty, such as a chronically ill or handicapped family member.

Quantifying adversity

After identifying what events or experiences have taken place, it is then necessary to accord some expression of magnitude to each experience, doing so independently of the individual's subjective response to it. In the original inventory method, each event carried a score, previously obtained by reference to a separate sample. This inventory approach has been further developed by many others, including Paykel *et al.* (1971), Tennant and Andrews (1976), and Henderson *et al.* (1981). In a useful review, Shrout (1981) has set out the theory, assumptions and strengths of the method compared to alternatives. The inventory approach assumes that a particular event carries the same impact for everyone, irrespective of the circumstances and independent of personality. It also assumes that respondents will be highly reliable in nominating the same item in the list for the same event, not omitting it or changing its category if they were asked to repeat the exercise after a few days. Yet we know this latter assumption cannot be made: people do change their choice of items for precisely the same event or experience (Steele *et al.* 1980; Neugebauer 1981).

Scales The issues to consider in scaling of life-events have been discussed by Shrout (1981). First, it is possible and indeed often sufficient, simply to make a count of the number of events endorsed, thereby according equal weight to each. Although contrary to our intuition, this surprisingly produces indices of adversity almost the same as when weighting is used, thereby avoiding the expensive preliminary exercise of determining weights for the population to be studied. But clearly it does violence to the intuitive notion that some events, such as death of one's child, are greatly more stressful than some trivial occurrence, such as losing one's purse. Furthermore, as Shrout suggests, to use weighted indices should add to the conceptual clarity of the effect of life-events on health. It is therefore usually desirable to find appropriate weights. These may be obtainable from the literature, but they may have to be established anew, as a subsidiary exercise, if the reference population differs markedly from the one being studied in attributes such as culture, age group or social class. Apart from personality, there are likely to be important systematic differences in what adverse events different groups experience in the first place, as well as their likely impact.

The work by Holmes and Rahe (1967) was based on the notion that life-events fall on a continuum of stressfulness; and that this continuum is itself the variable responsible for the onset of illness. They chose the amount of change or adaptation required of the organism by the event. They specified, wrongly as it turned out, that 'The emphasis is on change from the existing steady state and not on psychological meaning, emotion or social desirability' (Holmes and Rahe 1967, p. 217 and quoted by Shrout 1981). The list of 43 events was presented to a group of raters who were asked to scale them according to the amount of adjustment required. This is an exercise in *magnitude estimation* in which the following assumptions are made (Shrout 1981): (1) the continuum is so obvious that raters can place any event on it with certainty; (2) the scale values are universal, or at the very least are uniformly applicable within one population; (3) adaptation is the only important dimension relevant to disease aetiology; and (4) it is assumed that events or experiences can be placed on a ratio scale in the same way that psychophysicists measure perception of loudness or brightness. But perhaps we cannot say that one event is only half as stressful as another: sounds and life-events may not be equivalent in that way. Along with others (e.g. Brown 1981), we have to add that the weight assigned is unlikely to be valid across individuals: the impact of an event is likely to be significantly augmented or reduced by contextual factors in that individual's environment. It may therefore be misleading to accord the same weight to an event irrespective of the circumstances under which it was experienced. Clearly, an event such as 'miscarriage' can have very different impact, according to contextual factors and who is experiencing it.

The original Holmes and Rahe hypothesis about adaptation has not been upheld by the data. Instead, most workers now accept that it is the distressing quality of the event which has the stronger association with the onset of illness (Tennant and Andrews, 1978).

Reliability of the measure Whether the self-completed inventory or interview method is employed, it is highly desirable that the reliability of the information be determined. Attention to this has been scanty until recently (Neugebauer 1981). If retest and inter-observer reliability is low, any association which may exist with illness will be attenuated. The investigator should therefore assess reliability by having paired interviewers and by re-examining a subsample after a short interval, referring to the same calendar period of exposure (Steele *et al.* 1980). An index of reliability such as weighted kappa (Cohen 1968) which allows for raters agreeing only by chance, can then be computed. If it is low, the method for determining exposure to life-events will need to be improved. There has been only scanty attention to the validity with which people report life-events either in sickness or health. This is a fundamental deficiency which needs to be corrected.

Bias arising from symptoms

Persons with symptoms may report having had more adverse experiences than healthy persons, even if they have not. This was pointed out by Brown *et al.* (1973) and illustrates the phenomenon of 'effort after meaning', originally described by Bartlett (1932). Over-reporting of adversity could arise from the person's need to explain to himself and others the reason for his being ill; or from a gloomy outlook in keeping with depressed mood; or from the actual occurrence of events secondary to the illness itself, such as dismissal from work or disturbance of a personal relationship; and lastly, some of the earlier life-event inventories had items which unfortunately were more symptoms than life-events (e.g. 'difficulty in sleeping'). For these reasons, it can be hazardous to carry out cross-sectional studies of recent exposure to adversity in persons who are also currently symptomatic, if one wishes to throw light on disease aetiology.

One approach is to ignore any events which could have been generated by the illness or its prodromata, using only 'disease independent' events in the analysis. Many workers, however, believe that only prospective longitudinal designs can hope to advance understanding of the link between stress and illness. Here, it is necessary to distinguish between simple longitudinal studies in which *both* events and symptoms are measured at the same time on two or more occasions, and the much superior but more taxing strategy of measuring adversity when people are well, then re-examining them subsequently. The interval, however, must not be too great, lest any pathogenic effect be missed through its having been and gone before the second examination. The real problem is that any study of adversity, including a longitudinal design, is dependent on accounts of adversity after they have happened (Tennant 1983).

The context of the event

As Brown and his colleagues have argued (Brown and Harris 1978; Brown 1981), the impact of an event is partly determined by the social context; and by ignoring this, the inventory method is seriously misleading. He and his colleagues at Bedford College obtain exhaustive information about the personal and social context of each event or difficulty. By determining the circumstances, the interviewer is able to achieve a high level of empathic understanding of the experience, allowing a judgement to be made about its meaning for that individual, but deliberately *not* taking into consideration what the respondent reported having felt. Judgements about these events or difficulties, together with their severity rating, are later made by a trained team. In this way, the information used is interviewer-based, not respondent-based; and it is much more likely to reflect the actual experience of the individual, without carrying the serious methodological difficulties which arise when subjective responses are allowed to influence the judgement of severity. The Bedford College method is a unique contribution to epidemiology in that it allows both idiographic and nomothetic information to be combined.

Reaction to the event and personal vulnerability

The next issue in life-event research is the possible effects of the individual's personality (Henderson *et al.* 1981; Tennant 1983, 1985*a*; Perris 1984*a*, 1984*b*, *c*). First, certain personality types may recruit more adversity into their daily lives than do others. Although this is unarguably true of 'sociopathic' individuals, there is now the suggestion that persons high on the personality trait of neuroticism may also experience more adversity (Kiff 1981; Henderson *et al.* 1981, p. 186). A link between personality and life-events is a notion already described in general literature. The Orcadian writer, Eric Linklater (1934), has the main character in *Magnus Merriman* say, 'Nothing happens to a man except that which is intrinsically like him'. Secondly, it seems indisputable that the same adverse event or difficulty, even in equivalent social contexts, can have strikingly different effects on people. This may go some way to explain why only about 10 per cent of the variance in illness is explained by life-events, leaving most of it to other factors (Rabkin and Struening 1976); or why it is only a minority who do *not* adapt satisfactorily to major vicissitudes, such as death of a spouse or disaster (Clayton 1979, 1982; Raphael 1986).

The enduring intrapersonal characteristics of the individual, in attitudes and behaviour, may largely determine the response to environmental experience. And these same characteristics may be associated with other important factors in the causal model, such as social support. Hence it is incomplete to investigate the epidemiology of stressful experiences without at the same time considering personality attributes of the host.

Three personality traits are given here as examples likely to be important in aetiology: neuroticism, dependency, and self-esteem. Neuroticism, as a measure of reactivity of the nervous system (Eysenck and Eysenck 1964), has shown itself to be a powerful predictor of vulnerability to stressors, accounting in one prospective study for no less than 69 per cent of the variance in morbidity (Henderson *et al.* 1981, p. 186). But there may be serious problems due to confounding of neuroticism by symptoms themselves, particularily chronic ones (Katz and McGuffin 1987). Fergusson *et al.* (in press) have now provided important data on the issue, showing that neuroticism as measured by the EPI is largely a measure of chronic neurotic symptoms. Birtchnell (1984) has examined the trait of dependency as a vulnerability factor for depression. Self-esteem is now considered a personality trait of great relevance to vulnerability, but like neuroticism, its measurement is also open to contamination by depressive symptoms. A further psychological attribute which may be an important intervening variable, but which is not usually seen as a personality trait, is use of the mental mechanism of denial. The use of denial in some situations, by which individuals lessen the impact of experiences, has come to be seen as highly adaptive and successful, contrary to orthodox psychoanalytic teaching (Lazarus 1981). It is likely that these and other attributes account for much of the variability in the effect of adversity within populations. Outside extreme situations, the majority of people do not become ill after stressor experiences, although they may develop a number of transient symptoms.

The strength of the causal effect

Innumerable studies have shown an association between life-events and psychiatric morbidity on cross-sectional data. These have done little to advance understanding: they do not provide information about aetiology, but reiteratively confirm that persons with symptoms report more recent adversity than the healthy. Yet there are many reasons why this might be, other than a causal effect. To infer the latter, it is necessary to use a prospective longitudinal design, whereby the exposure to adversity is assessed before the onset of symptoms. Even then, a positive association may conceivably be due to the prodromata of the illness, or to personality traits which predispose both to adverse experiences and psychiatric disorder.

The strength of the association may be expressed as the amount of variance, in a continuous measure of morbidity, which is 'explained' by the life-event score in a multiple regression analysis. This has been found to be only about 10 per cent, even in prospective studies (Rabkin and Struening 1976), which means that about 90 per cent of the variance remains unaccounted. But an alternative expression for the contribution to aetiology is the relative risk statistic (see also Chapter 2, p. 16). This is the ratio of the incidence of a particular disorder in those exposed and those not exposed. Paykel (1978) reported relative risks, estimated as approximations from retrospective data, of between 2 and 7 for psychiatric disorders in the six months following exposure to high adversity. In a recent prospective study of London women, Brown *et al.* (1986*a*) have reported data on the incidence of depression, from which a relative risk of 14 can be calculated for women exposed to a provoking agent. This indicates a powerful pathogenic effect in this sample. For statistical reasons, such relative risks are quite compatible with as little as 10 per cent of the variance being explained.

Unresolved issues

Which method? Choosing between the inventory and the interview method deserves careful consideration, according to the purpose of the study and the resources available. The inventory has the strength of being brief, taking about 15 minutes if performed with care, either by self-completion or by being read to the respondent. It requires very little training of the examiner, and there is no time-consuming rating session with skilled research staff afterwards. It is therefore cheap to use. It does produce information on exposure to adversity, and at the same time it spares the respondent for enquiry into other important material, such as symptoms, past history, personality, parental style, and current social environment, without tiring him or reducing the completion rate in a survey. But as we have seen, the inventory method does not enable actual experiences to be reliably allocated to particular items on the list, so that respondents may place the same event under different headings, thereby attracting different scores. The placing of the event in time may also be unreliable and no contextual factors are considered. Finally, the use of ratio scales for measuring adversity is open to dispute. These defects are so serious that, in our view, simple inventory methods are not to be recommended. Too often, the information they produce may be gravely misleading.

The interview method developed by Brown and his colleagues requires careful training for both the conduct of the interview and the subsequent rating of events. There have been some studies making a formal comparison of the two methods. Bebbington *et al.* (1984) made the important observation that a simple inventory instrument (Tennant and Andrews 1976) failed to describe 5 per cent of 'marked' events and 21 per cent of 'moderate' ones. The relative risk of minor psychiatric disorder associated with preceding events was 3·1 for those identified by the Brown method, but only 1·4 for those using the inventory. The extra labour and cost involved is very appreciable, but justified.

How specific is the pathogenic effect? Recent work suggests that fairly specific associations may exist between type of life-event and the type of illness which follows. Finlay-Jones and Brown (1981) have produced evidence for a link between losses and the onset of depression; and between threatening events and the onset of anxiety states. On the other hand, it seems likely that for the same event or experience, some individuals will develop psychological symptoms, while others will have mainly physical consequences. The operative factor here may be as much a diathesis typical of the individual, rather than some characteristic of the event. This issue calls for clarification. It certainly seems prudent to consider the onset of both psychological and physical symptoms after exposure to adversity, rather than to focus on only one group of disorders. That is, a case can be made for being prepared to identify a range of morbidity following adversity, rather than being prepared to recognize only affective or other psychological symptoms. (Andrews and Tennant 1978*b*)

Cross-cultural comparisons

Although some work has been accomplished in this field, it remains a promising area for further study of human adaptability and coping. In many communities of the world, the death of children and young persons is a familiar event, as is extreme poverty, natural disaster, and the threat of starvation. Life-event ratings in such populations must be immeasurably higher than in the more familiar samples from materially affluent nations. But it has yet to be demonstrated that the incidence of morbidity related to such stress is significantly greater in less developed countries. One reasonable hypothesis is that an important variable is the baseline of adversity for a population. What may be pathogenic is the level of adversity experienced above this baseline. This leads directly to the desirability of having a measure of the average level of adversity being experienced in the study population, then comparing that to the level in high risk groups. As we have seen before, reference to the denominator and to the baseline experiences of its members is a necessary step in trying to identify pathological processes.

The clinical significance of life-events

Much of the foregoing has been about efforts to measure, then to determine the effects of stressful experiences. To the earlier investigators in the 1960s and 1970s, there was the hope that life-events would explain much of the aetiology of illness, particularly mental disorders; and that this might be a promising road to prevention. Instead, as Andrews and Tennant (1978*a*) have pointed out, these initial hopes began to fade, and instead a preoccupation with method emerged. There are indeed some very considerable technical problems in measuring exposure to stressful experiences, but it is essential to keep the real objective in mind: to determine the role of adversity in the onset of illness, or of relapse.

Finlay-Jones (1988) has set out a succinct review of the evidence. Life-events involving a loss, he concludes, are an important cause of depressive illness and its outcome, of suicidal behaviour, and possibly of mania. Where life-events involve danger, there is some evidence that they cause the onset of anxiety states. The general review by Tennant (1983) considered only prospective studies, where any causal effect of life-events can be more clearly delineated without contamination by symptoms. He was forced to conclude from these prospective studies that the 'findings overall do not seem to show that life-events have any substantial causal role in neurotic illness'. He advocated more emphasis on prospective designs, more sensitive measures of stress with short follow-up periods to 'catch' the pathogenic effect, and the inclusion of personality measures.

The role of life-events in the onset of depression has been reviewed in some detail by Bebbington (1985). The central task has been to interpret the evidence from many studies that adversity precedes the onset of depression or depressive symptoms. There is some evidence that the association may be stronger for mild states than the more severe ones familiar in clinical practice; and that when events do lead to depression, they take place two to three months before onset. This fits with the contrast made by Birley and Brown (1968) and Brown and Birley (1968) between the 'formative' effect of events in depression and their triggering effect in schizophrenia. As life-events do not invariably lead to morbidity, the role of vulnerability has come to be recognized as of crucial importance. Such vulnerability may be social, intrapersonal, or biological.

Much attention has been paid to vulnerability factors for depression. Brown and Harris (1978) reported four from their Camberwell data: loss of mother before age 11, not working outside the home, lack of a confiding relationship with a husband or boyfriend, and having three or more children aged under 15 at home. The interpretation of these findings has been disputed, the argument mainly being about demonstration of interaction effects (Tennant and Bebbington 1978; Bebbington 1980). The important consequence of this work is that investigators no longer seek a simple association between adversity and morbidity, but recognize that other sets of variables coact with adversity. A causal model, therefore, whether in research or in individual case-work, has to be much more elaborate. Figure 4.2 is a useful starting point for this purpose. It shows some of the sets of variables which may contribute to symptom onset (in this case, depression); and how these variables are themselves inter-related. Bebbington (1985, 1988) has cautioned that causal models which hold for relatively mild affective disturbances, as met in surveys, may not hold for the more severe disorders seen in clinical practice.

In a collaborative study between a social psychiatry and a psychiatric genetics team, the relationship between adverse experiences and familial aggregation of depression has now been investigated (Bebbington *et al.* 1988; McGuffin *et al.* 1988). From preliminary analyses, McGuffin and his colleagues report no significant difference in the risk of depression in the first degree relatives of patients whose illness was associated with adversity, compared to the relatives of patients whose depression was not. These authors then

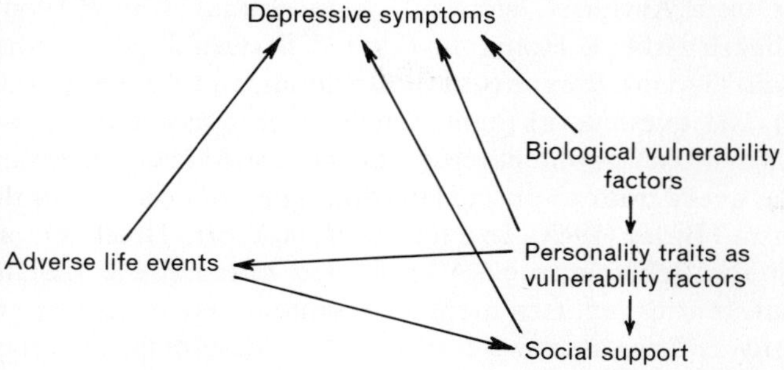

Fig. 4.2. Adversity and depressive disorder: a simplified model.

compared first degree relatives of depressives with a community sample from the same part of London (Bebbington *et al.* 1981*a*), and found that more of the relatives were cases *currently* of depression than in the community (19 per cent as against 9 per cent). But they also found that more relatives had experienced recent threatening life-events (21 per cent as against 7 per cent). This has suggested to these workers that event-associated depression occurs in hazard-prone and not just stress-prone persons. Life-events as well as depression show familial aggregation. This may account in part for the well-known *association* between adversity and depression.

For life-events and schizophrenia, a review by Tennant (1985*b*) sets out the evidence. He was led to conclude that life-events may precipitate hospital admission of schizophrenic patients; that events may be associated with affective or neurotic symptoms in schizophrenia; and that there may be some association between life-events and expressed emotion, leading to relapse. Tennant found the evidence that adversity contributes to the *onset* of schizophrenia was less conclusive, with only the study by Brown and Birley (1968) having the methodological strengths to support this. It showed a likely causal effect from independent life-events in the three-week period before onset. Leff *et al.* (1983) have reported that independent life-events contribute to relapse in patients already diagnosed as having had schizophrenia and coming from families with high expressed emotion. The findings of a cross-cultural study of life-events and acute schizophrenia throw new light on the subject. This work was carried out by investigators in seven countries under the auspices of the World Health Organization (Day *et al.* 1987). The centres were Aarhus (Denmark), Agra (India), Cali (Colombia), Chandigarh (India), Honolulu (United States), Ibadan (Nigeria), Nagasaki (Japan), Prague (Czechoslovakia), and Rochester (United States). The investigators found that life-events may contribute to the onset of acute schizophrenic episodes and tended to cluster in the two to three weeks prior to onset. This finding is congruent with that of Brown and Birley (1968). In a review of the World Health Organization Study, Bebbington (1987*b*) pointed out that the Indian and Nigerian centres reported more very acute onsets of schizophrenia, yet many of these cases were unrelated to life-events. This suggests that the acute but relatively benign psychoses seen in developing countries may not be psychogenic.

EXTREME EXPERIENCES

Whereas every individual receives a scattering of life-events in the course of daily life, only a few are exposed to extreme experiences in the course of a lifetime. In the 20th century, the Nazi Holocaust is the most recent example in the Western world, and has been extensively documented in psychiatric research (Eitinger 1964). Information is sadly lacking on the mental health consequences of similar Holocausts in Indo-China and Africa. There is overwhelming evidence that concentration camp experiences induce chronic mental ill-health lasting 40 or more years later. Tennant *et al.* (1986*a*) found increased rates for depression 40 years later in Australian servicemen who had survived extremely harsh treatment, including forced labour, humiliation, torture, and starvation, on the Burma Railway and in Changi Prison under the Japanese. Despite having had these extreme experiences, a small number of persons were found to have been spared any psychiatric sequelae; and a few have been reported to have had their coping abilities enhanced by the experience (see also Tennant *et al*, 1986*b*).

Staying well under adversity

Antonovsky *et al.* (1971), in an important paper on this issue, examined the question of why a not-inconsiderable number of camp survivors are well-adapted, despite their extreme experiences. It is unclear if this group represents one extreme of a normal distribution, or if they are numerically larger forming a distinct and important category. These authors suggest three possible factors: an initial underlying strength, a helpful environment after the experience, and a 'hardening' process which allows the survivor 'to view current stress with some equanimity'. In all of this, it has to be borne in mind that those available for psychiatric examination are a tiny proportion of all those who were exposed; and they are clearly a survival élite from amongst the latter. But as there is no doubt, or indeed surprise, about the pathogenicity of extreme experiences, it is surely as useful to investigate why some individuals are not adversely affected. This is likely to be a fertile avenue for treatment and prevention.

The importance of the previous personality and of effective coping styles is now emerging as a consistent theme. Henderson and Bostock (1975, 1977) studied seven men who survived in a raft at sea without food for 13 days after shipwreck. Although five of the seven had developed substantial psychiatric disorder at follow-up one year later, one man claimed to have been enriched by the experience, seeing himself as more resourceful and having more enjoyment from his marriage and family.

Helzer *et al.* (1979) and Helzer (1981) investigated the incidence of depression in American servicemen who had fought in Vietnam. Their examination was carried out two to three years after the men's return. They compared them with a group who had been eligible to be called up, but were not. They found greater morbidity for depressive symptoms in the veterans, but this difference diminished after controlling the pre-service variables. They then compared combatants and non-combatants within the veteran group, recognizing that some pre-Vietnam characteristics could have predicted both combat assignment and later depression. They did find higher depression in the combatants, but pre-service differences seemed to play a much stronger role than in-service variables. The depressive symptoms, furthermore, were of short duration. In further analyses of the data, Helzer (1981) showed that as servicemen were exposed to increasing levels of combat stress, the increase in depressive symptoms was much less in those who did not have pre-service vulnerability factors. These included social deviance in childhood or adolescence, drug use, failure to graduate from high school, alcohol abuse, parental arrest, and parental psychiatric problems.

A comprehensive account of the psychodynamics and social psychiatry of disaster has been given by Raphael (1986). In a study of persons exposed to a natural disaster in the form of a large bushfire in Australia, McFarlane and Raphael (1984) and McFarlane (1985, 1986) have reported the pattern of symptoms and their time-course.

McFarlane went on to consider vulnerability factors. He found that intense exposure to the bushfire disaster was characteristic of persons with post-traumatic stress disorder. Constitutional factors, however, were prominent in his series, acting alongside the level of exposure, the perceived threat or loss, and intercurrent life-events.

The implication from those observations is that even when exposure to adversity is extreme, constitutional factors contribute importantly along with other social and experiential variables in determining who will develop a mental disorder. Each of the above studies is a reminder that even in persons exposed to extreme stresses, morbidity is induced in only a minority, and pre-exposure attributes of the individual are apparently more important than the level of stress in predicting who will develop symptoms. This conclusion is essentially the same as that proposed by Slater (1943) and Slater and Slater (1944) on the basis of observations made on UK servicemen during the Second World War.

BEREAVEMENT

The death of a spouse, child, or parent is generally taken to be amongst the most stressful of life-events, although they are clearly both universal and phylogenetically ancient experiences. A considerable literature has accumulated on the consequences of bereavement for physical and mental health. Excellent reviews have been conducted by Klerman and Izen (1977) for the former; and by Clayton (1974) and Raphael (1983) for the latter. Bereavement, like physical trauma, has obviously been experienced throughout human evolution, so that it is not surprising that restitutive mechanisms have developed.

The emotional and behavioural responses to bereavement have now been repeatedly documented. Early classic papers were those of Lindemann (1944) followed by Clayton (1974, 1979), Maddison and Viola (1968), and Parkes (1970). The stages of grief are essentially the impact itself, a period of mourning with depressive affect, and the recovery phase.

Mortality

If the experience of bereavement has an impact on the organism, the most extreme consequence would be an increase in mortality. There is epidemiological evidence that an increase does indeed take place, although there are some conflicting findings, such as those of Clayton (1974) where no excess was found. She has suggested that the evidence points to an increase in mortality only in men over age 55 (Clayton 1982). Klerman and Izen (1977) reviewed the evidence to conclude that the hypothesis for increased mortality was indeed supported. They noted a trend for greater risk in the younger bereaved, and a peak of mortality in the second six months after bereavement. These authors have considered the possible mechanisms whereby mortality could be increased. Kraus and Lilienfeld (1959) and Young *et al.* (1963) proposed homogamy (unfit marrying unfit), common infection, shared exposure to health-impairing factors, loss of care after bereavement, and biological changes due to the effect of grief on physiological systems. Bartrop and Porritt (1988) have examined critically the evidence that the stress of bereavement alters the immune system.

Physical health

In their exhaustive review, Klerman and Izen (1977) considered a large number of studies reporting increased morbidity from cancer, heart disease and infections. As they point out, methodological defects have been frequent in this work, including absence of control groups and a failure to control for age or other confounding variables. But overall, there does seem to be an increased incidence of physical illness (Kraus and Lilienfeld 1959).

Psychiatric morbidity

This has been well reviewed by Clayton (1982). In the year following bereavement, depressive symptoms are common, particularly in the first few months. There is an increase in the symptoms of sleep disturbance, feeling someone is to blame, and feeling both hopeless and worthless. But some depressive symptoms are rare: suicidal thoughts, retardation, and pervasive guilt. Severe anniversary reactions are unusual and are associated with a poor prognosis. Admission to psychiatric care was found by Stein and Susser (1969) to be increased in widows during the first 12 months of bereavement, but not later. They pointed out that admission may not be due to bereavement itself, but to the diminution in care it brings for persons who would otherwise have managed to remain in the community. Clayton (1982) concluded from her review that the relationship between bereavement and reaching psychiatric consultation is not at all consistent in the literature; and that psychiatric hospitalization is exceptional.

In an important controlled study of a random sample of widowed persons, Clayton (1974) found not only an absence of increased mortality, but no difference in the use of medical services, despite the presence of more depressive symptoms in the bereaved group. The latter also used more hypnotics. Other studies have consistently reported an increased use of alcohol, tobacco, and medication (Clayton, 1982).

The majority of the bereaved recover their mental health within a few months, and certainly most do so within a year. Raphael (1983) has provided a detailed account of factors influencing outcome. The best predictors are good physical or mental health prior to the bereavement. In this way, the findings are consistent with those on persons exposed to extreme experiences.

UNEMPLOYMENT

The rise in national unemployment rates in many Western countries is a social phenomenon now of great relevance to psychiatry. It has become a priority that knowledge be obtained about the effect of unemployment on mental health and the implications for treatment and prevention. Research on this subject has been of high quality, with a clear appreciation of the variables at play, in addition to the primary ones of mental health and the state of being unemployed. Warr and Jackson (1985) have set out the major issues in their account of a prospective study of 629 unemployed working-class men. Other useful studies are those by Eisenberg and Lazarsfeld (1938), Cohn (1978), Banks and Jackson (1982), and Feather and Barber (1983).

There is a definite association between being unemployed and impairment of mental health, particularly with depressive symptoms. But on top of this, there are many other factors which have to be considered if the association is to be more fully understood. In a group of persons who have become unemployed, it cannot always be assumed that their mental health was unimpaired prior to unemployment. In some circumstances, it could be that persons with chronic depression or other psychological impairment may be more likely to lose their jobs. But this is clearly irrelevant to many contemporary conditions, when either loss of a job or failure to obtain one is often independent of the individual.

The age group being considered is important, because several studies have shown that the middle-aged are the most affected by symptoms, compared to younger or older persons. There seems to be a tendency for symptoms to increase over the first three months, then to level off. Commitment to employment is an important variable, Warr and Jackson (1985) having proposed that it may help in coping to become inured to the prospect of a prolonged period without paid work. This may modify self-perceptions, allowing the individual to predict and plan the future more realistically. Financial stress is clearly a central issue for many, particularly those with dependents. Previously existing medical conditions tend to worsen, at least subjectively, as the period of unemployment lengthens. For many, the worst period psychologically is within the first few months, when many additional life-events arrive in the train of being unemployed: financial problems, a very different daily routine, different domestic and social interaction, and the need to deal with official benefit agencies. Adaptation to this new role takes some months.

Jackson and Warr (1987) have shown that in communities with longstanding, high unemployment rates, unemployed men have lower rates of neurotic symptoms than in communities with only moderate or low unemployment. This difference held after allowing for personal factors known to be associated with mental health during unemployment (age, length of unemployment, family composition, and the importance of paid employment). Jackson and Warr argue that this finding suggests communities with high unemployment have certain characteristics which give rise to better mental health in unemployed men. They point out, however, that the material deprivation in such areas is associated with poorer physical health and premature death; and that unemployment remains associated with impaired mental health, even in these more sympathetic environments.

Much of the research on unemployment has used self-completion instruments such as the General Health Questionnaire (GHQ) to measure psychological symptoms. Unless it is scored by the method of Goodchild and Duncan-Jones (1985) which takes the response 'no worse than usual' as positive for those symptoms which can be chronic, the GHQ is known to produce false negatives amongst persons with chronic symptoms. It is also possible that a self-report instrument may generate more false positives in such a group, through the social expectation that they will not be as well as when in paid employment. For these reasons, a standardized interview such as the Present State Examination (PSE) or the Diagnostic Interview Schedule (DIS) is advisable in research on this group, at least in a subsample. The PSE was used in a two-phase design by Finlay-Jones and Eckhardt (1984) in a sample of 401 unemployed persons aged 16–24 years in Canberra. They found a remarkably high case rate of 49 per cent, based on the Index of Definition.

In examining a cohort of unemployed persons, one should bear in mind that a selection effect may have taken place, whereby those who are mentally well may have a higher probability of rejoining the workforce. This could lead to a relative excess of symptomatic persons in the remaining members of the cohort. Finally, there is good evidence from longitudinal studies (e.g. Warr and Jackson 1985) that being re-employed has a beneficial effect on mental health. This is surely an important piece of information, both for treatment strategies in psychiatry and for government policies.

SOCIAL SUPPORT

Whereas the environment is the source of many noxious influences, it may also include some beneficial elements. An intuitively appealing hypothesis is that human relationships may have a protective effect against adversity. The 16th century essayist Francis Bacon (1965) put the notion concisely in his essay 'On friendship'. He wrote:

> . . . this communicating of a man's self to his friend works two contrary effects; for it redoubleth joys, and cutteth griefs in halfs. For there is no man that imparteth his joys to his friends, but he joyeth the more; and no man that imparteth his griefs to his friends, but he grieveth the less.

The implication is that, in the course of social relationships, particularly where these are emotionally close, something beneficial is conveyed from one person to another. Though only in the last decade, this idea has now been quite intensively investigated in relation to mental health, to physical morbidity, and to mortality.

The hypotheses

Care should be taken to distinguish between at least three separate hypotheses about social support. These are: that it has a direct and independent effect in its own right on mental and/or physical health, whether or not adversity is also present; that it provides a buffer or cushioning effect against stress, but has no independent effect in its absence; or that in persons who have already developed affective or neurotic symptoms, it has a therapeutic effect, shortening the episode and reducing symptoms. So far, most attention has been paid to the first two of these. We now examine their origin.

Ethologists have pointed out that interaction with other members of the same species has played an important part throughout primate evolution (Hamburg, 1968*a*, 1968*b*), so that the presence of close others may have become an essential element in the environment for adaptive behaviour to be maintained. In another discipline, sociologists have extended the work of the first social scientist to examine social ties and social support, Emile Durkheim (1897). Research on social networks has shown how these are organized and what structural features are to be found universally (Cooley 1909; Faris 1932; Barnes 1954; Litwak and Szelenyi 1969). At the same period, also following the work of Durkheim, psychiatric epidemiologists began to enquire into the link between social disorganization and mental disorder (D. C. Leighton *et al.* 1963*a*). Maslow (1968) argued that after food and shelter, a basic human need was to engage in relationships. From this confluence of ideas, it can be readily understood how Cassel (1976) came to formulate the stress-buffering hypothesis in his celebrated paper, 'The contribution of the social environment to host resistance'.

The idea has held considerable appeal for both epidemiologists and social scientists. It is a hypothesis which proposes an aetiological factor outside the individual, in his social environment. Such a paradigm has long been a mainstay of social psychiatry, with its emphasis on extrapersonal factors as major determinants of mental disorders. But in addition, the social support hypothesis has some special attractions peculiar to it: its confirmation could provide a rationale for treatment or even for prevention, including primary prevention; and it has appeal within the politics of health and social services. Research on social support has become a growth area, not only within the mental health field but also in general medical epidemiology. There are now several reports of reduced morbidity or mortality in persons with plentiful social support (Nuckolls *et al.* 1972; Berkman and Syme 1979; Berkman 1986). Detailed reviews of the field have been provided by Greenblatt *et al.* (1982) and Broadhead *et al.* (1983). For psychiatric disorders, Henderson (1984), Schradle and Dougher (1985), and Alloway and Bebbington (1987) have examined the evidence so far available.

What should be measured?

Although it is a convenient term for daily use by health workers or helping agencies, social support is a label for something which has many components. In the course of relationships with other persons, an individual both receives and provides a number of things. Just what these are proves very difficult to articulate. There are obvious items, such as the provision of essential goods. Then there are services to others, such as food preparation, grooming, or child-minding. But after that, one enters the affective or psychological domain and the conceptual task is harder. A debt is owed to R. S. Weiss (1974, 1979, 1982) who attempted to set out what he conveniently termed 'the provisions of social relationships'. He proposed that there were at least six: attachment, social integration, an opportunity for nurturing others, reassurance of personal worth, a sense of reliable alliance, and obtaining help and guidance from others in facing difficulties. These are not easy constructs to measure, but together they are likely to capture most of the ingredients whose existence is implied in the every-day term 'social support'. Another typology of social support is by Kahn and Antonucci (1980). Theirs has the attraction of being a mnemonic with the three headings: affect (someone expressing affection), affirmation (someone saying they are of a like mind), and aid (help and advice). It also has the merit of conforming to the well-established triad of affect, cognition, and behaviour.

We know of four approaches to the measurement of social support. First is the use of sociodemographic variables as coarse indicators of relationships. A second method is to construct a scale based on a small number of questionnaire items enquiring about marital status, living arrangements, contact with others at work, in the neighbourhood and at home, and involvement in group or community activities. A third method has been to focus mainly on one type of social relationship. Because affectionally close or intimate ties have been expected to carry the most aetiological significance, it is these which are likely to be chosen for scrutiny. This has been done with great thoroughness by Brown and his colleagues in determining the presence of a confiding relationship in women (Brown *et al.* 1975, 1986*a*; Brown and Harris 1978). Their Self Evaluation and Social Support interview (SESS) (Brown *et al.* 1986*a*) is particularly successful in establishing whether or not the respondent (in Brown's work always a woman) has an affectionally close relationship. A particular strength is that it is interviewer-based rather than respondent-based, and thereby is less contaminated by subjective perception.

Brown *et al.* (1986*a*) have recently extended their assessment of a relationship to determine *post hoc* what quality of support was *actually provided* by the confidant when the respondent was faced with adversity. They refer to this as 'crisis support'. Although such data are very open to distorted reporting, particularly by a respondent who has developed symptoms of anxiety or depression, the attempt to find out what actually happened in the person's hour of need is commendable. Determining what crisis support was obtained carries the same difficulty as information on life-events: both have to be obtained at some time after they were experienced; and special attention is accorded to those persons who had poor crisis support and now have symptoms.

A fourth approach has been the construction of instruments for measuring a range of social ties, together with what they provide for the respondent. Examples are the interview developed by McCallister and Fischer (1978), the Social Support Questionnaire by Sarason *et al.* (1983), the Interview Schedule for Social Interaction (ISSI) (Duncan-Jones 1981*a*, *b*; Henderson *et al.* 1980, 1981) and the Social Support Network Inventory by Flaherty *et al.* (1983). The ISSI has now been used in English, German, Swedish, Hebrew, and Hindi. Instruments of this type carry the advantage that they set out to examine many facets of the complex called social relationships. Their deficiency may be that they are respondent-based and thereby open to a number of distortions in reporting; and that they do not sufficiently explore the actual support received and the promotion of self-esteem this brings.

Reliability has been shown to be satisfactory for this type of instrument. In their validation, problems have arisen. The availability of particular categories of relationship and what they provide for the respondent can be confirmed, at least to some extent, by interviewing an informant. But it is much more difficult to validate the true quality of the relationship. If there is a marked discrepancy between the respondent's own assessment of the support and some external judgement, the interpretation is unclear.

Herein lies one of the main issues in weighing the evidence on social support: are the measures a valid reflection of the actual social environment, or are they confounded by personality factors, which inevitably must influence how that environment is construed, or possibly even constructed, by the individual? Whether or not a person has good social support is not necessarily a piece of information exclusively about that individual's social environment: it may also be an index of personality, in so far as this enables him or her to establish, then to maintain, relationships with other persons. That is, intrapsychic factors may to some extent determine a person's social environment. In this field, psychiatric epidemiology once again faces the distinct possibility that there are important interaction effects between environmental and intrapsychic variables. To ignore one or the other can give only an incomplete picture.

The evidence

Mortality There is now impressive evidence for an association between good social ties and reduced mortality, with at least four studies leading to consistent findings (Berkman 1986). The association seems to be stronger in men and in some social or ethnic groups. The manner in which the effect is mediated is not at all understood. It is conceivable that certain personality traits may confer both longevity and a rich personal network. This is an area of considerable interest.

Mental disorders It is fairly well established that persons with depression and neurotic disorders presenting in psychiatric outpatient clinics have fewer close relationships and reduced personal networks (e.g. Henderson *et al.* 1978*a*, *b*; Brugha *et al.* 1982). The most likely explanation is that social withdrawal is an important symptom of depression. Yet the restricted network may have predated the depressive illness. There might also be a nosocomial effect along the lines of Berkson's bias (Berkson 1946), in which a combination of neurosis and lack of social support leads preferentially to receiving professional help, compared to persons who have only a neurosis (see Chapter 2, p. 12). Because of the implications for both treatment and prevention, this area offers some attractive prospects for further useful research.

For persons at the general population level, there are a number of cross-sectional studies, mostly showing an association in the expected direction. But these provide inadequate evidence for the hypothesis because the information on social support has invariably been obtained from persons who also have psychiatric symptoms. Two studies with prospective longitudinal designs have produced findings which are in conflict (Henderson *et al.* 1981; Brown *et al.* 1986*a*, *b*). These authors have collaborated in examining the possible reasons for the differences (Henderson and Brown, 1988 (*vide infra*)).

In the Canberra study, an association was found between social support perceived as inadequate by the individual, and the subsequent onset of neurotic symptoms *under adversity*. The elements in the social support measure included both close ties or attachments and more diffuse relationships. It was perceived inadequacy of social support, not its reported availability, which had some predictive power. But the association was not strong in contrast to the measure of neuroticism, which accounted for as much as 69 per cent of the variance in subsequent symptoms. As we noted before, however, it has to be acknowledged that measures of neuroticism are likely to be contaminated by subclinical symptoms, thereby inflating the apparent association.

The study in Islington by Brown *et al.* (1986*a*, *b*) was based on a sample of some 400 working-class women. For those who were married, troubled interaction in the marriage, measured at time 1, predicted later onset of depression at the case level. For single mothers, lack of active emotional support from another similarly conferred vulnerability to breakdown. Brown and his colleagues took their investigation an important further step by determining at follow-up what support was actually received by those faced with a severe event. In this way, they tried retrospectively to find out if the support obtained was in keeping with the woman's original account of her social resources. Women who were 'let down' in their time of need had a particularly high rate of onset of depression. The Islington study also included measures of self-esteem in the first interview. Negative evaluation of self was a strong predictor of later depression in those exposed to stressors. But this effect was greatly reduced if the woman did receive crisis support.

The Canberra and Islington studies differ in a number of important ways, which may explain their different findings. These include the sociodemographic characteristics of the two populations, the samples used, the measures of psychiatric disorder, the measures of social support, and of personality. These issues and their significance have been discussed critically by Henderson and Brown (1988) in a paper which looks for possible causes of the different findings. The latter author considers that there is now sound evidence for a protective effect from social support obtained from a close confidant; both authors believe that intrapersonal attributes need to be studied further for their role both in forming the person's social environment and in predisposing towards minor psychiatric disorder.

Conclusion

The place of social support in protecting against psychiatric disorders can be set out as follows:

1. Social support has many components.
2. It is not yet clear which of these components are effective in protecting against stressors.
3. Crisis support may be only weakly predicted by reports of longer-term availability.
4. The types of psychiatric disorder against which social support is active are not yet known. Neurotic depression, anxiety neurosis, and mixed neurotic states including somatic complaints, are likely candidates.
5. A crucial distinction should be made between the support actually available to a person, and his or her perception of its adequacy.
6. This leads to the important issue of personality, which may be an intervening variable: persons with certain personality traits may, on the one hand, have deficient relationships; and on the other, a vulnerability to depressive disorder.
7. Any demonstrably protective effect of social support may not be uniform across social groups: that is, support may be more effective in some than others.
8. The impressive evidence on reduced risk of mortality suggests that social support may indeed have a biological effect in reducing the effects of stressors.
9. The bulk of the research done so far has been on the aetiological role of support. Much less is known about its therapeutic effect in those who already have psychiatric symptoms, and for whom an augmentation of social support may be tried prescriptively. Such a trial was conducted by Parker and Barnett (1987) on highly anxious primiparous mothers. They compared the effect of extra support from professionals, and from lay sources with a control group, using the ISSI to measure any changes in the mothers'

personal networks over a period of 12 months. They found that anxiety was reduced in the professional intervention group, but the ISSI scores remained unchanged. This finding points to our lack of understanding of the relationship between social support and the relief of minor psychiatric symptoms.

5

The social consequences of mental disorder

(1) Consequences for the person: impairment, disability, and handicap; relevance to clinical practice; disabilities due to mental disorder; effect of psychiatric disorder on living conditions; recruitment of adversity; the primary group. (2) Consequences for the family: as a whole; effects on the child; on the parents; on the spouse. (3) Economic consequences. The costs of schizophrenia. Forensic psychiatry.

We have seen how the social environment contributes to the onset and course of mental disorders, but it can also be affected by them. In this chapter, the social environment becomes the dependent variable. Psychiatric disorders are then one of many variables influencing the social life and conditions of individuals. A good source for further reading and references on this important subject is the volume edited by Robins *et al.* (1980) entitled *The social consequences of psychiatric illness*. A useful framework of thinking about the subject is to consider the effect of *specific* psychiatric disorders, first on the person and secondly on the family; then to examine the wider economic consequences for the individual and for the state. We shall discuss this topic under these three general headings.

1. CONSEQUENCES FOR THE PERSON

Disability

As with physical symptoms, the emergence of psychiatric symptoms may be accompanied by impairment of function in daily life. But here one has to be careful to avoid confused reasoning about the nature of mental disorders: some of the symptoms and signs themselves refer to impairment in role performance, such as irritability or social withdrawal. There is therefore some overlap between the two sets of variables: symptoms and impairments. But it is also reasonable to hold that having a disease or disorder may lead to impairment as something separate and secondary. In an important publication, the *International classification of impairment, disabilities and handicaps*: *A manual of classification relating to the consequences of disease* (WHO,

1980), the following sequence underlying illness-related phenomena has been set out, together with definitions:

Disease–Impairment–Disability–Handicap

This schema and its terms have proved very useful in practice. *Impairment* is disturbance of structure or function at the organ level. *Disability* is the consequence of impairment, in terms of functional performance and activity by the afflicted individual. It represents disturbance at the level of the person. *Handicap* is concerned with the disadvantages experienced by the individual as a result of impairments and disabilities. It reflects disturbance to the ways in which the person interacts with the surroundings, or is able to adapt to them.

Mental disorders, like physical illness, cause impairments, disabilities, and handicaps. Although this is self-evident, it is only quite recently that each of these has been related to specific psychiatric disorders such as major depression or schizophrenia. J. E. Cooper (1980) has set out a framework for describing and classifying social disability. De Jong *et al.* (1985) have tackled the specific issue of social disability in schizophrenic patients. The World Health Organization has now developed an instrument, the Psychological Impairments Rating Schedule (PIRS) and has undertaken a collaborative study on impairments and disabilities associated with schizophrenic disorders (WHO 1979; Jablensky *et al.* 1980). Sartorius *et al.* (1986) have reported on the two-year outcome in 1379 persons in different cultures, finding a more favourable prognosis in less industrialized societies. As part of that study, J. E. Cooper and Bostock (1988) found that the relationship between schizophrenic symptoms and impairment is by no means straightforward, and is not at all as one might have expected. It seems that people vary considerably in the impairment that results from superficially similar symptoms and in how they react to the symptoms and their social circumstances. Furthermore, social disability can persist *in the absence of psychotic symptoms*. These observations correspond to the concept of the social breakdown syndrome developed by Gruenberg (1974), in which he described the social concomitants of severe psychiatric disorder, their likely origins, and strategies for their prevention. (See also Gruenberg and Kennedy, 1988.)

Relevance to clinical practice

Attention to disability in severe mental disorder has immediate relevance to the assessment and management of patients. It is not enough to consider only the symptoms. There should also be emphasis on how the individual is functioning in daily life, within the family, at work, and in the wider social context. It seems increasingly clear that a linear relationship may not always operate between symptoms and such social impairment. What additional factors are at play is not at all clear. In the individual patient, attributes worth particular attention are social and personal assets. It is helpful to be able to recognize these resources, then to harness them in the plan of management. As an example, Wing (1966) noted how well patients' initial attitudes to their difficulties predicted outcome in an Industrial Rehabilitation Unit. Most clinicians and nurses are aware that some people remain likeable, despite severe disorder and severe disability. They thereby tend to fare better, both in interaction with others in hospital and in re-establishing their lives outside. Such features are perhaps particularly apparent in the elderly.

This leads logically to a second area: how those around respond to the illness and behave towards the patient. The practical benefits of exploring this are considerable. Some behaviours may be helpful, whereas others can reinforce maladaptive patterns in the patient. Still others may be directly pathogenic, as with strong *expressed emotion*, leading to increased likelihood of relapse in schizophrenia, depression, and possibly other disorders. (See Chapter 7, p. 148.)

Disabilities due to mental disorders

(i) Disabilities In assessing what disabilities are present in a person with a particular psychiatric disorder, it is useful to employ the classification set out in the World Health Organization Manual, where the following categories are defined (WHO 1980, p. 144 *et seq.*): behavioural changes; body disposition; communication; dexterity; personal care; situational; and locomotor. As an example, an elderly person with a dementia is likely to have behavioural disabilities in terms of self-awareness, orientation, personal safety, occupation, and the way he or she conducts himself within the family. Dysphasia and impaired comprehension will hinder communication, while personal care will be affected. Similarly, a patient with a marked depression is likely to communicate less, to pay less attention to others, to have diminished interest in self-care and to be unable to cope with some social situations. A person with agoraphobia has principally a situational disability, in that there is reduced tolerance

of certain environments. Readers will find that this World Health Organization classification is, in a number of instances, insufficiently differentiated to take account of the disabilities occurring in some common psychiatric syndromes. But for particular projects, this can readily be rectified by constructing supplementary measures for the purpose in hand.

(ii) Handicaps The areas of handicap specified in the World Health Organization Classification are: orientation; social integration; physical independence; economic self-sufficiency; mobility; other handicaps; occupation. The manual provides rating scales with a definition for each level. The scales for occupational and social functioning are particularly relevant. Handicap in the occupational role is assessed on a 10-point scale with clear rules for assignment. For example, a rating of '2' (curtailed occupation) would be accorded to a depressed mother of young children who is experiencing difficulty in running the household and caring for the children, although she is still managing. If substantial help were needed from others, her rating would increase to '3' (adjusted occupation). The scale for impairment in social integration is also clearly of particular relevance in clinical psychiatry. A 10-point scale covers the range from full social integration to the alienated or isolated. For some purposes, it would certainly be necessary to focus in more detail on social performance in marriage, and on the quality of interaction with parents, offspring, and others in the individual's personal network; and to determine what changes have taken place since the onset of the illness. For these purposes, an interview with a third party or informant is usually needed.

Effects of psychiatric disorder on living conditions

When a person becomes psychiatrically disturbed, this may have a considerable influence on where he comes to live and with whom he is in contact in daily life. This almost certainly goes a long way to explain the ecological findings of Faris and Dunham (1939, 1960) in their classic work on the concentration of cases of schizophrenia in the central area of Chicago. The cases had probably drifted there as their disorder progressed. In her study of the elderly in San Francisco, Lowenthal (1964, 1965) obtained clear evidence that mental disorders led to changes in social conditions and living patterns. In a field survey of the elderly in Mannheim, B. Cooper and Sosna (1980) found that persons with organic states were strikingly absent amongst those living alone. These authors justifiably suggested that a combination of biological and social handicaps is so disabling that a high proportion of such persons are admitted to institutional care at an early stage in their disorder. This process is clearly likely to be most operative where the afflicted person has no other caretaker in the household. When B. Cooper and Sosna went on to examine the amount of social contact in their community sample, they found that severe isolation was not more marked in the mentally ill; milder forms of isolation were present in those with affective and neurotic conditions. Significantly, they found that contact with social services was very infrequent in the overall sample; and that not one of the 42 mentally ill persons was under psychiatric treatment. In Hobart, Australia, Kay *et al.* (1985) and Henderson *et al.* (1986*a*, *b*) surveyed the elderly living at home. They found that older persons had fewer social relationships than younger adults, but were more content with what they did have. As in B. Cooper and Sosna's finding, elderly persons with either depression or cognitive impairment had less social interaction than the mentally healthy.

In a survey which included both a 5 per cent random sample of the elderly residents in the community and coverage of those from the same population currently in institutional care (mainly nursing homes), B. Cooper (1984) found that only 10 per cent of all psychiatric cases and only one-fifth of those with psychoses (mainly dementia) were in any form of institutional care. This and other studies have consistently shown that most elderly persons with severe psychiatric disability are still living in the community, usually in a household with other persons. We shall return below to the implications of this for the family.

Recruitment of adversity by persons with mental disorders

Whereas life-events play a role in the *onset* of many disorders in adulthood, including psychiatric illness, some important questions remain about the relationship. For most research purposes, it is customary to consider only those life-events which are judged to be independent of the disorder or its possible prodromata. This leaves still open the possibility that some individuals attract, or even elicit, more life-events than others; and that a proportion of such persons may also have a vulnerability to specific psychiatric disorders. Such propositions are not often made in social psychiatry and epidemiological research, although they are very familiar to clinicians, particularly psychotherapists. This is an instance where the aetiological models used by research and clinical groups have drifted too far apart. Dohrenwend and Dohrenwend (1980) and Kreitman (1980) proposed that not only do some persons have greater vulnerability to develop psychiatric symptoms under stress, but some are also more prone to experience these stresses. Henderson *et al.* (1981) noted an association in a community sample between the neuroticism score and reported exposure to subsequent life-events. The evidence is not entirely satisfactory as yet, because of the possibility of biased reporting, and difficulties in obtaining measures of personality uncontaminated by symptoms, but it is prudent for social psychiatry to recognize that a person's social environment and experiences are not entirely independent of that individual's own attitudes and behaviour. People are to some extent the architects of their social environment. The density of adverse life-events may be greater in some persons with mental disorders. This may be due in part to their premorbid personality, and in part to the social consequences of the psychiatric disorder itself. As we noted in Chapter 4, McGuffin *et al.* (1988) have evidence that exposure to adversity is in part familial.

There are some implications arising from this for clinical practice: it is likely to be helpful if practitioners work with the patients and family to reduce the density of life-events, as the continuing impact of these may play an important part in bringing about relapse or chronicity of symptoms. How such a reduction can be achieved is far from clear. Indeed, in comparison with the abundance of research on life-events, how to reduce them or their impact has not been studied with as much vigour. This is an area of preventive psychiatry which now deserves to be expanded.

The patient's primary group

The primary group is a term introduced by the sociologist Cooley (1909) to refer to those in a person's social world with whom there is both interaction and commitment. The term personal network is better retained to refer to those with whom there is only interaction. Personal networks are therefore numerically larger than primary groups. In the case of minor psychiatric disorder such as neurotic depression and anxiety states, there is some evidence that the primary group is reduced in size and in the quality of interaction. One of the first demonstrations of this was by Miller and Ingham (1976) in

Edinburgh. They confirmed the observation of Brown *et al.* (1975) that depressed women tend to lack a close confiding relationship, but found that amongst persons consulting a general practitioner for psychological symptoms, there was also a reduction in more casual, less intimate friendships. A similar pattern was found by Silberfeld (1978) in Toronto.

In a case-control study of persons referred for neurotic complaints to a psychiatric service (Henderson *et al.* 1978*b*), the cases were found to have spent the same amount of time with their primary group, but more of that time had been affectively unpleasant. Cases had fewer attachment figures, nearly a half reporting that they had only one. The majority considered that their principal attachment figure gave them less support than they needed. Cases also had fewer good friends and fewer social contacts outside the household. This study was later replicated by Brugha *et al.* (1982) in Dublin, using a similar source of patients and the same Social Interaction Schedule. They found very similar results for neurotic patients, but not for those with retarded depressions.

In depression, Blazer (1983) found that elderly persons identified in a community survey actually had had an *increase* in their social interaction when followed up 13 months later. This could suggest that psychiatric disorders may have a care-eliciting consequence in some circumstances. In an earlier paper entitled 'Care-eliciting behavior in man', the present author proposed that behaviours associated with many psychiatric states may elicit increased care and concern from others; and that these disorders may have a higher incidence in persons who perceive themselves to be conspicuously lacking in such care and concern from important others (Henderson 1974). By having a care-eliciting effect, the symptoms and behaviour may go some way to correct the perceived deficiency, although at some social and personal cost. This is well-illustrated in many cases of para-suicide, neurotic depression, and the abnormal illness behaviours which are so common in general practice and hospitals (Pilowsky 1978, 1988).

For other psychiatric disorders, there is, so far, even less information on social relationships and the temporal sequencing of changes in its composition. For schizophrenia, it seems likely that the primary group is often reduced premorbidly, and that the onset of the psychosis diminishes it further (Henderson 1980). The extensive studies of Brown *et al.* (1958, 1962, 1966) and Wing and his colleagues

(Wing *et al.* 1964; Wing 1978*a*) have been directed expressly at the social world of the patient with already established schizophrenia. Furthermore, this body of work has examined the effect of the social environment on the subsequent course of the disorder, rather than the effect of schizophrenia on the primary group. We shall return to the former in Chapter 7, because of its considerable importance for theoretical development and for services.

An issue of the *Schizophrenia Bulletin* (Vol. 4, 1978) was largely devoted to social networks in this diagnostic group. Morin and Seidman (1986) claim that the personal networks of 'revolving-door' patients are characterized by being inflexible and unstable. They have advocated that the personal network is a desirable focus for intervention. A review of the subject leads to the conclusion that personal networks, not surprisingly, are impaired in schizophrenia, but that the really important question is what that observation implies for social care (Henderson 1980). Does repair of the personal network do good or harm? And under contemporary conditions, in which many mental hospitals are being closed as a policy, what is the effect on their discharged inhabitants of having a major change in their primary group? It is here that the work on Expressed Emotion (EE) is so relevant, because it has helped to clarify what elements are pathogenic within the patient's primary group.

2. CONSEQUENCES FOR THE FAMILY

The family as a whole

For the consequences to families of having a mentally ill member, we shall firstly consider what is known about the overall impact, then deal with effects specifically on children, parents, and spouses. The subject has been reviewed by Fadden *et al.* (1987*a*), to which we shall refer below. There is also the development of family therapy as a sub-speciality (e.g. Bentovim 1986; Bloch and Crouch 1985). An early but influential study by Clausen and Yarrow (1955) provided a detailed analysis of the impact on 33 families of having a schizophrenic member. These workers reconstructed the nature and size of the stresses on family members from the time schizophrenic symptoms first appeared. Many further studies have since followed, often prompted by the recent enthusiasm for a shift to community care. The majority have focused on severe mental disorders, such as that by Pasamanick *et al.* (1967) on the families of 226 schizophrenics treated in the community. In their volume *Schizophrenia at home*, Creer and Wing (1974) gave a comprehensive account of the social and interpersonal impact of this disorder. The personal experiences of persons who have lived with a psychotic family member have been published by the National Schizophrenia Fellowship in the United Kingdom (Wing 1975).

In their celebrated study comparing a community care service in Chichester with a mental hospital based service in Salisbury, United Kingdom, Grad and Sainsbury (1966*a*, *b*, 1968) were able to examine the impact on families of the whole range of mental disorders across all adult age groups. Their account is worth reading in detail. With a two-year follow-up assessment of the effect on families, they found that all measures pointed to a greater burden in the community care group. But this did not apply to those families who had been under the greatest burden at the time of referral: they were helped equally by both services. When Grad and Sainsbury explored their data to identify who was contributing most to family burden in the community service, they found these tended to be younger, mainly neurotic patients who, although not a severe burden, continued to cause their families problems.

Arey and Warheit (1980) have reviewed the literature on the 'psychosocial cost of living with psychologically disturbed family members' and presented findings from their own work. The evidence is impressive that stressor effects exist, and that these are often present over long periods of time. But as Kreitman (1980) points out in his review of their paper, it is unwise to neglect the methodological hazards in such research. Family members who are already anxious or depressed may readily ascribe their state to the behaviour of others; and if one person in the household is psychiatrically unwell, he or she may be the butt for such an explanation. Furthermore, in assessing clinical series, one should bear in mind that only a small proportion of all morbidity reaches psychiatric services; and distress in relatives may be one important factor in the patient's referral. Clinical series, therefore, have a high probability of having an over-representation of symptomatic relatives who report a considerable subjective burden, and go on to seek professional help. We may less often see those families who have a comparable burden, but may not experience as much distress, and do not reach specialist services.

The review by Fadden *et al.* (1987*a*) has considered the essential issues which constitute the burden, and points to the neglected matter of helping relatives to cope. Fadden and her colleagues have tried to clarify the concept of burden. It means that one or more in the household is doing 'more than their fair share', has activities restricted outside the relationship, and experiences a greater or lesser degree of distress. Platt (1985) has examined the methods for measuring burden and the difficulties encountered. Financial difficulties are often substantial as part of the consequences of having an ill family member. The attitudes of relatives to the illness and the sick member are an important aspect, because they are often painful. They include anger, resentment, guilt, and seeing the patient as weak-willed. They are also an entry point for helpful interventions. The symptoms and behaviour which are most burdensome are now well-established. They include those which endanger the patient's safety or that of others; disturbed nights; incontinence; and 'negative' or excessively withdrawn behaviour. Repetitive questioning or hypochondriacal statements can be extremely wearisome. It is notable that overtly violent or socially embarrassing behaviours may not be those which cause the greatest burden.

Although clinicians must be aware of the burden placed on relatives by patients' symptoms, they have not shown great interest in helping families, with few exceptions. Wing (1982) pointed out that, unlike professionals, relatives have no special training in dealing with difficult behaviour, they are on duty all the time, and their relationship with the patient makes it difficult to remain neutral, and not to become emotionally involved.

There is evidence, reviewed by Fadden and her colleagues, that professionals (mainly psychiatrists) often behave unhelpfully toward relatives seeking guidance, and hold prejudiced attitudes about what constitutes 'good' or 'bad' relatives. These issues have become particularly relevant at a time when community care is being widely advocated. Fadden *et al.* (1987*b*) have extended our knowledge in this field by conducting a study specifically of burden to relatives of patients with depressive disorder.

There is good evidence that interventions are effective, as in schizophrenia (Brown *et al.* 1962; Vaughn and Leff 1976); and in depression (Hooley 1986). A number of further studies are currently being conducted, in which relatives are offered training programmes in how to behave and how to cope. For example, Dr Henry Brodaty and his colleagues in Sydney have for some time now been conducting a training service for the relatives of elderly persons with dementia, who care for these persons at home. The results of this and similar pilot programmes suggest that there are benefits for the relatives' mental health. In some disorders, of course, such as schizophrenia, there are well-established benefits also for the patient. Kuipers and Bebbington (1988) have provided an explicit guide for the relatives of persons with severe affective disorder or schizophrenia. They address the whole issue of living with the mentally ill, how to help the patient, and how to protect one's own mental health.

Effects on the child

Having a sick parent is a risk factor for psychiatric morbidity in children. A major contribution to this field has been by Rutter (1966). Since that publication, many leads have been pursued in what is clearly a deserving area. Rutter found that psychiatric morbidity, in the form of neurotic states and conduct disorders, was increased in children where one parent had a mental disorder, but the effect was also apparent with chronic physical illnesses in a parent. He has now provided a review of the evidence which has accumulated since his 1966 publication, together with a bibliography (Rutter 1987). He has emphasized the need to understand the *mechanism* for the association if preventive action is to follow. In summary, the increased risk for psychiatric disorder carried by children of sick parents is mediated in the following ways: through genetic transmission, through biological and physical effects on the fetus, and through the family environment.

The genetic effects do not seem specific. Raised rates for psychiatric disorder in the children have been found for parental schizophrenia, depression, alcoholism, and personality disorder, but the morbidity is heterogeneous.

There are now well-established adverse effects on the foetus from maternal alcoholism and smoking. Alcohol is cytotoxic in the first 10 weeks of pregnancy, causing a deficiency in brain growth. Further effects on neural cells take place later in pregnancy. These teratogenic properties of alcohol lead to the fetal alcohol syndrome, characterized by mental retardation and cranio-facial malformation. For opioids, the evidence suggests that children are at increased risk for psychiatric disorders, but that this is more likely to be due to poor maternal functioning rather than a direct effect of the drug on the fetus.

The family environment has now been shown consistently in many studies to have an important effect on the mental health of children. Rutter's (1966) earlier work had suggested that the risk was greater when parental symptoms directly affected or involved the children. Such direct impact took place, for example, when a psychotic parent's delusions referred to the child, or when the child had to take part in some obsessional rituals of the parent. Rutter and Quinton's (1984) prospective study of parents with psychiatric disorder now shows that such situations are exceptional. Instead, the most common pathogenic influence is exposure to hostile or aggressive behaviour by the parent. The effect of family discord as a risk factor is likely to be determined by its strength and frequency. Regarding family break-up, Rutter concludes that what probably matters most is not the child's separation from parents, but the multiple stresses associated with it, and the family discord which precedes and follows the child's entry to alternative care.

Rutter concludes that in treating parents with a mental disorder, clinicians need to be on the lookout for three things: the extent to which the disorder is associated with family discord, negative feelings towards any of the children, and impairments of parenting. He points out that the evidence firmly contradicts the view that young children are not aware of parental tensions and conflict. Parents need to be helped to reduce their hostilities, to avoid conflicts impinging on their children, and to improve their functioning as parents. The non-ill parent may need to be encouraged to take on more of the day-to-day care of the children. In the specific situation of a puerperal psychosis, much too little is known about the desirability of having the mother continue to care for her baby. Rutter rightly declares that we do not yet know that babies do *not* suffer from exposure to severely ill mothers.

Individual differences in children's responses In his review, Rutter (1987) considered the remarkable variability in the response of children to having a mentally ill parent. Less than half develop any psychiatric disturbance. The characteristics and context of the parent's illness play an important part in determining the likelihood of morbidity in the children. This is reduced if the parent's mental disorder is mild, brief, and not associated with family discord and conflict, impaired parenting or break-up. But attributes of the child also play an important role. Boys have an increased vulnerability for reasons which are not yet at all clear. Parents may be more likely to engage in conflict in front of sons than daughters. Boys tend to respond to conflict with aggressive behaviour and girls with emotional distress. This may lead in turn, Rutter suggests, to boys' receiving more direct criticism, which may further compound the difficulties which they are having to handle. Temperamental differences in either sex are likely to be important determinants of morbidity in children. Protective factors include a good relationship with one or both parents prior to the parental illness, having an emotionally supportive non-ill parent, a best friend, robust self-esteem, and a repertoire of problem-solving abilities.

Rutter specifies three points in the application of this knowledge to clinical practice with mentally ill parents. First, it is important to focus on how children are actually responding, rather than on reports by the parents or others. Secondly, attention should be paid to the pattern of parent–child interaction, to learn how the child has been responding, and how both the parents have responded in turn. Thirdly, the clinician should be concerned with the family as a whole, including its other kin and family friends. The family is to be recognized as a positive resource, for which there is usually no satisfactory substitute. Rutter ends his review with the challenge that the knowledge now available has considerable implications for policy and for practice, but data are lacking on the extent to which preventive action is effective.

Effects on parents

As a specific field of enquiry, this subject is strikingly underexplored. If a child or adolescent has a long-lasting psychiatric disorder, this clearly will be a chronic stressor of some magnitude to the parents and to other siblings, grandparents and family. The impact will depend on many factors: the nature of the disorder itself, the abnormalities of behaviour it brings to homelife, the social and personal resources of the other family members, the quality of the relationship between the parents themselves, and the quality of their premorbid relationship with the young person.

Most clinicians are familiar with the distress, guilt, self-questioning and resentment which arise in parents whose child has developed conditions such as a depressive illness, behaviour disorder, psychosis, or drug dependency. Little is known yet about the patterns of such parental reactions, their consequences for family life and marriage, and their longer-term outcome. Not infrequently, the parents themselves may have some constitutional vulnerability which further compounds the picture, as when one parent is prone to depression or alcohol abuse.

The best information so far refers to the impact on families of having a severely mentally retarded child at home. In a study of considerable significance, Dupont (1980, 1986) examined this in detail in 39 such families in Denmark. She found that on average they spent seven hours a day, seven days per week in the care, supervision, occupation, and training of the severely retarded children. For 80 per cent of her series, the parents' sleep was disturbed. Only one-quarter of the children could be left alone, and then only for about half an hour. Cultural activities were restricted for 87 per cent, 77 per cent had limited contact with friends, and 59 per cent had given up going on holidays. In two-thirds of the families, siblings took a substantial part in the care of the child. In Dunedin, New Zealand, Romans-Clarkson *et al.* (1986) investigated the mental health and social relationships of the parents of 54 children with major physical or mental handicap, compared to 184 controls. They found that caring for a handicapped child has great impact on the mental health of mothers, but less on the fathers. Interestingly, the size and quality of the mothers' personal networks were not different from the mothers of normal children.

Whereas some psychiatric disorders, in contrast to mental retardation, may place rather fewer physical and time demands on parents, there is good reason to believe that psychological stresses may be even more marked; and that general freedom of family life may be severely limited. The area is a rich one for exploration, and the knowledge gained could be put to good use in helping such families. It is likely that mothers, in particular, carry major burdens. Wilkin (1979) has expressed it concisely: 'Community care does not mean care by the community, nor does it mean care by the family. It means maternal care with varying but generally low levels of support from others'.

Effects on the spouse

The spouses of persons with neurosis have been studied much more thoroughly than the spouses of persons with other categories of disorder. Kreitman (1964) compared 75 neurotic patients and 95 matched controls, finding that patients' spouses were higher in neuroticism and had more physical and psychological symptoms than same-sex controls. As the duration of marriage progressed, neuroticism scores in the spouses of neurotic patients increased; and psychological symptoms also increased in prevalence. Furthermore, the correlation between spouses' scores for neuroticism was found to increase with duration of marriage in the patient pairs; but it decreased in the controls. Kreitman concluded that neither assortative mating nor interaction between marriage partners could explain his findings. He noted that in the neurotic patients' marriages, interaction was considerably more isolated than in the controls. He found differences in the amount of social activity, patients and their spouses having less interaction with others outside the family.

Kreitman *et al.* (1970) subsequently went on to examine the social integration of couples where one spouse had a neurotic illness or character disorder. They found support for the hypotheses that, compared to normal couples: (1) patients' marriages are characterized by more time in face-to-face contact; and (2) the wives of male patients have less diversity of social contacts and poorer social integration. These findings were obtained by use of a time-budget. Kreitman noted a progressive increase in social activity in normal wives as their marriage progressed, but no such increase in patients' wives. There are likely to be diagnosis-specific differences in such patterns of marriage. Presumably, the impact is greater where symptoms in a spouse are chronic, rather than only occasionally present as in a recurrent affective disorder.

These findings strongly suggest that neurotic disorder in a spouse has an adverse effect on the other; and that it also can considerably restrict social interaction outside the home, an activity which itself may carry benefits for mental health.

ECONOMIC CONSEQUENCES

There is good reason to believe that psychiatric disorders bring about a rather greater cost both to family incomes and to national exchequers than is generally appreciated. Neurosis or depression is a commonly cited reason for premature retirement from the civil service in several Western countries. It is certainly related to absenteeism in industry. We shall now consider the financial cost of schizophrenia, as one psychiatric disorder for which good data recently have been obtained.

The costs of schizophrenia

Studies of the costs associated with schizophrenia provide a powerful illustration of the economic consequences of only one, albeit a major mental disorder. Over a decade ago, Gunderson and Mosher (1975) estimated an annual direct cost in the United States of between US$11·6 and $19·5 billion. The lower of these two estimates amounted to no less than 2 per cent of the gross national product for 1975. In a searching analysis of the financial costs in schizophrenia, Andrews *et al.* (1985) calculated that the 1975 expenditure in the United States was about US$208 000 per case. They went on to make a painstaking comparison of the costs of schizophrenia and myocardial infarction in New South Wales, Australia. Total annual costs were US$139 million and US$295 million respectively: the total cost for schizophrenia is about half that of myocardial infarction. By contrast, the cost per case was US$131 333 for schizophrenia but only US$22 626 for myocardial infarction, for, although the latter has an incidence 12 times greater than schizophrenia, schizophrenia costs six times as much *per case* as myocardial infarction. Andrews and his colleagues then determined that the national funding in Australia for research into schizophrenia in 1982 was only one-fourteenth that spent on myocardial infarction. They concluded that current practices and policies for funding research were 'not producing the rapid growth in knowledge that might have been expected to follow Kraepelin and Bleuler's delineation of the disorder 70 years ago'. Indeed, it is rare in any area of medical and behavioural science for either expenditure or research effort to be well matched to public health needs.

FORENSIC PSYCHIATRY

'Forensic psychiatry is simply the application of general psychiatry to people who are in one way or another involved in the legal process' (Gunn 1979). As a subspeciality, it is presently undergoing considerable expansion, with the need for it being increasingly expressed in the judicial system, in hospitals, prisons, youth services, and health authorities. Contrary to popular belief, forensic psychiatry is not concerned solely with violence, as Gunn's definition should make clear. It is considered in this chapter because of its obvious social relevance. More detailed accounts can be found in Gunn (1979, 1982,

1986) and in the report by a World Health Organization working group (WHO 1977). The principal issues are the relationship between mental disorder and crime, the management of violence, the concept of responsibility, and research and training in forensic psychiatry.

The first of these is of particular relevance to psychiatric epidemiology. It is most clearly depicted as a Venn diagram where the components are psychiatric disorder, criminal acts, prisons, and mental hospitals (Fig. 5.1).

The diagram refers to persons. For a country or a community, it is possible to estimate the number of persons with psychiatric disorders, including those disabled by severe disorders of personality; and to determine the number of persons in psychiatric wards or hospitals, and the number of persons in prisons. But it is not possible to estimate the numbers carrying out criminal acts during the same time period, but who are not discovered, let alone also found guilty. Here, all we have at best is the number of persons coming before courts, some of whom are found guilty. To the writer's knowledge, there is no available estimate of the prevalence of psychiatric disorder in this latter population, and there obviously can never be one for the much greater population of persons who have committed crimes but not been prosecuted (not shown in Fig. 5.1).

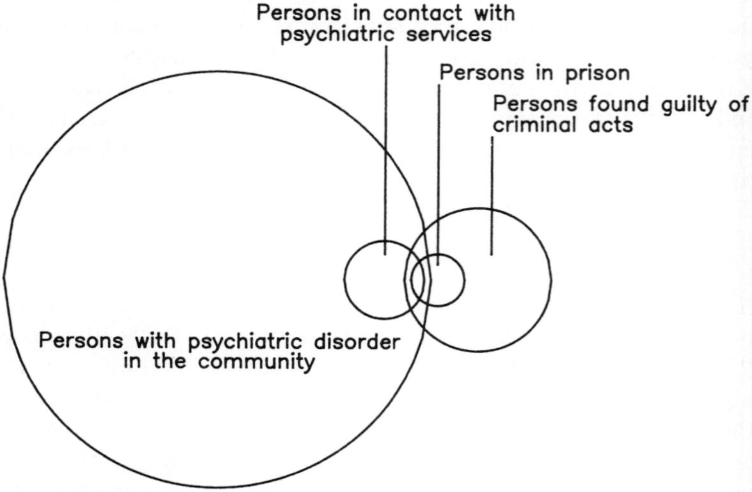

Fig. 5.1 A Venn diagram of forensic psychiatry. (Note: not drawn to scale, see text.)

Gunn (1979) reports that 31 per cent of persons in prisons can be regarded as psychiatric cases. When we ask what proportion of psychiatric patients have carried out a crime in, say, the previous 12 months, there are no available data. Gunn cites a study by Guze and his colleagues who found what appears to be a lifetime prevalence of 4 per cent in a series of 500 psychiatric patients. This is unlikely to be higher than the general population. The reader will see that, once again, the epidemiological approach which asks 'What is the true denominator out of which this group is derived?', opens up a new perspective on some of the fundamental issues in forensic psychiatry.

Concerning violence, there is no sound evidence that psychiatric patients are more violent than the general population. Gunn has set out a framework for clinical use in evaluating violent behaviour in a person, and its appropriate management in different contexts. In many countries at present, there is a re-examination of policy about secure units for persons likely to continue to be violent.

Because of its social relevance, forensic psychiatry is now clearly an area of growth, one where training has become an important part of the development of young psychiatrists and other mental health workers. It is also one where research opportunities abound. Here, epidemiological data are likely to be particularly useful. Readers might consider the many questions which are raised by entering forensic psychiatry as one of the column headings in Tables 3.1 and 3.2. To this agenda have to be added a number of issues of essentially a social nature, about which information and experience are much needed. These include the impact of criminal acts on spouses and families, the effect on them of imprisonment, the social environment in prisons and remand centres, and the social component of prevention in forensic psychiatry.

6

Mental disorders and primary care

Psychiatric morbidity which reaches primary care; determinants of seeking help; psychiatric morbidity recognized by general practitioners; the reduction of hidden psychiatric morbidity; screening; training general practitioners; some studies of primary care; classification; social work and primary care; clinical psychology; future prospects.

PSYCHIATRIC MORBIDITY WHICH REACHES PRIMARY CARE

When people experience psychological symptoms which they or their families find unmanageable, a universal practice is to seek help from a professional. In most countries, including some of the poorest, this takes place at a general practitioner's surgery or local health clinic. The pioneering work on psychiatric disorders in primary care was carried out by Shepherd and his colleagues in London general practices (Kessel 1960; Shepherd *et al.* 1966, 1981). They examined the psychiatric morbidity which general practitioners recognized, the characteristics of the patients, and what treatment they received. The understanding gained from these studies has since been extended in important ways, notably by Goldberg and his collaborators (Goldberg and Blackwell 1970; Goldberg 1972; Goldberg and Huxley 1980; Bridges and Goldberg 1985). Although this body of work refers specifically to service conditions in Britain, it is likely that the same general principles operate in many other countries, particularly those where general practice services are a prominent part of health care. Collectively, this work has shown what proportion of primary care patients have a psychiatric disorder, how these disorders are presented, and what factors determine their recognition and adequate treatment. This subject is clearly central to the delivery of basic mental health care. A concise review has been set out by Shepherd (1983), and a useful collection of essays and reviews are in an edited volume by Shepherd *et al.* (1986).

In this chapter, there are three principal issues to consider, because together they encompass all aspects of the role played by the family physician in the care of persons with psychiatric disorders. These are:

1. The process by which people reach their doctor and are then recognized, or not recognized, to have psychiatric symptoms.
2. The kinds of symptoms or syndromes which typically present before family physicians.
3. The response of the doctor, the treatment or management subsequently undertaken, and the outcome.

A concise account of each of these issues has been given in an important book by Goldberg and Huxley (1980). The field it covers has special relevance for the trainee in the mental health professions, at a stage when he or she is coming to appreciate the great range of psychological and behavioural pathology, and the extent to which individual practitioners come to be familiar with different sectors in that range. What is useful is that the perspective which Goldberg and Huxley provide is epidemiological: it represents mental disorders as these occur in the general population; and it estimates what proportion reach primary care or specialist clinics. This perspective is salutory for the younger clinician, who may come to believe that the profile of mental disorders as they present in the clinic is a true reflection of all that occur. But psychiatrists, as we shall see, have direct contact with only a small fraction of the whole, albeit the most severe or the most disabled. For understandable reasons their experience of mental disorders is usually limited to only those persons they treat in clinics, hospitals, and out-patient departments. But the universe of persons with mental disorders is much wider. Many obtain care from other professionals, or informally from resources within their own personal networks. But general practice is the main setting in which persons with symptoms of psychological origin present.

A central issue here is the concept of a case, to which we have already referred in an earlier chapter (p. 26). This is a man-made construct, imposed by setting a threshold on what is a continuum of symptom severity. In the primary care setting, a threshold originally derived from mental hospital practice may not be appropriate, either for identifying or classifying the cases encountered. Perhaps too many of the basic assumptions in psychiatry have been forged in hospitals or in psychiatrists' consulting rooms; the profile of

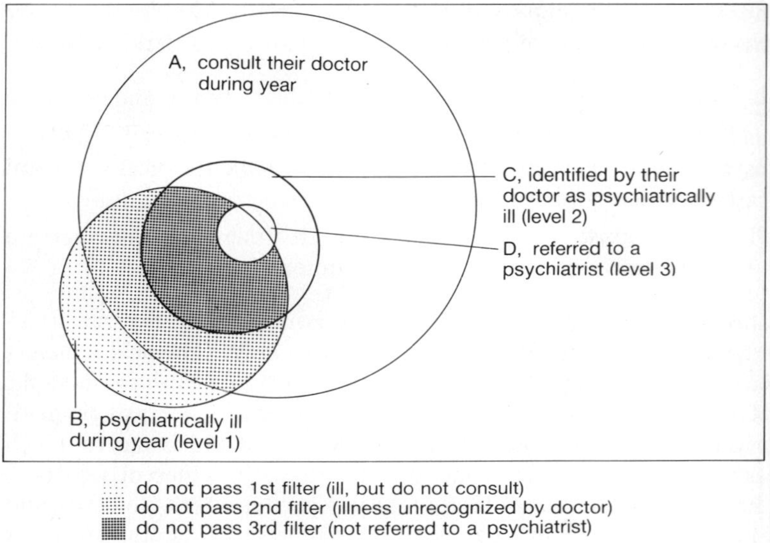

Fig. 6.1 A Venn diagram of psychiatric disorders and primary care. (From D. Goldberg and P. Huxley, 1980. *Mental illness in the community*. Tavistock Publications, London. Reproduced with kind permission of the authors and publisher.)

morbidity in these latter settings is not representative of psychiatric disorders as they really occur in the general population; nor is it necessarily valid when applied to patients at the primary care level.

Goldberg and Huxley (1980, p. 13) have constructed a Venn diagram which conveniently summarizes a great deal of information. We have reproduced it here (Fig. 6.1). It is drawn to scale, so that the proportions represent the distribution of psychiatric disorders as they really occur at each level of care. In this way, it relates the reader's clinical work to the overall presentation of morbidity; and it has the capacity to stimulate important questions on the relationships between the groups of patients represented by different circles.

The outer square is the general population being considered, and is therefore the denominator out of which all other groups have their origin. It will usually have geographical boundaries; and there should be a statement about whether or not it includes children, the elderly, or persons living in special circumstances, such as the homeless, nursing home residents, those in residential schools or hostels, hospitals, and prisons.

The largest circle, A, represents all those in the population who have consulted their family doctor at least once in a given period, usually one year, for any complaint, whether it be physical or psychological. We can count only those doing so for the first time in say, six months, so that we are dealing only with new (and treated) episodes. Circle B defines those who developed a psychiatric disorder in the course of one year. Goldberg and Huxley have introduced the term *level 1 morbidity* to refer to that group. At this point, readers should be alerted that, for convenience, a categorical binary state has now been imposed on our thinking. People are being rated as either ill (cases) or not ill. But psychiatric morbidity is often best seen as dimensional. So we have had to force a cutting point on each syndrome to define who is a case, and who is not. Note that circle B is not entirely within A: some people have a psychiatric disorder but do not consult their doctor. Goldberg and Huxley (1980, p. 45) suggest that this number is usually quite small, at least in industrialized countries where medical care is free for the consulter, and for persons whose symptoms are at the case level, as the latter is conceptualized by psychiatrists.

DETERMINANTS OF SEEKING HELP: THE FIRST FILTER

Some persons at level 1 morbidity will seek professional help, although not all will. This is what Goldberg and Huxley refer to as the *1st filter*. Although the severity of a symptom is clearly one major factor impelling persons to go to their doctor, there are other significant determinants. This is the subject of illness behaviour, as developed by Mechanic (1978). It can be defined as the manner in which 'symptoms may be differentially perceived, evaluated, and acted (or not acted) upon by different kinds of persons' (Mechanic 1962). It is a key concept for social psychiatry. For psychological symptoms, Ingham and Miller (1976) investigated the 1st filter in a Scottish general practice, finding that problems or symptoms other than the psychological ones probably precipitated the consultation, although severity of the target symptom and its recency of onset both played an important part. In a key paper reviewing the subject, they have drawn attention to the following influential factors (Ingham and Miller 1982): how disruptive to life or incapacitating the symptom is;

the distress it causes; its rapidity of onset; concomitant adverse life-events; sex and age; the influence of other adults; and personality traits such as intropunitiveness. Each of these has some effect. At least for psychological symptoms, adverse events do seem to influence the decision to consult a general practitioner. In women compared to men, there is not only a higher base rate for symptoms at the general population level, but they have more severe symptoms, or are more willing to acknowledge their existence (see also Chapter 3, p. 37, *et seq.*). In addition, women may be more ready to go to the doctor when they fall ill. Consultation rates steadily increase from the teens to old age. Prompts from other adults, particularly spouses, may be an important influence in the decision to consult, although little is known about this. Finally, the more the number of symptoms, the more likely the person will seek help. In all of the above, the dependent variable under consideration is the individual consultation. There is an important distinction to be made between this and the *frequency* of consultations, which is influenced by other factors.

THE PRESENTATION OF PSYCHIATRIC DISORDERS AMONGST PRIMARY CARE CONSULTERS

This is *level 2 morbidity* in the Goldberg and Huxley terminology. It refers to those consulters who have a psychiatric disorder and who have passed the 1st filter. Their general practitioner may or may not have detected the illness. In Fig. 6.1, this group is shown as the stipled area inside circle A. Goldberg and Huxley call the *2nd filter* those factors which inhibit doctors (or other primary care staff) from recognizing that a psychiatric disorder is present. Notice in Fig. 6.1 that a few persons are so identified who do not in fact have a psychiatric disorder. But the issue calling for most attention in the psychiatry of general practice is what can make the 2nd filter most permeable, whereby general practitioners can be competent at recognizing those who have psychiatric disorders and who, in addition, have taken the step of consulting them.

Patients will by no means always speak of their symptoms in words which clearly signal their psychological nature. The language may be vague, such as ‘feeling run down’, followed by some somatic complaints. This seems to be a common pattern both in Western and other cultures. It is not only in Northern Europe and North America that psychiatric morbidity is presented in predominantly somatic language. Somatization should not be considered as a diagnostic category in its own right. Instead, it is a common psychological mechanism, defined by Kleinman and Kleinman (1985) as 'the expression of personal and social distress in an idiom of bodily complaints with medical help-seeking' (quoted in Bridges and Goldberg 1985; see also Kleinman 1986). This is the manner in which many people experience affective symptoms; but it is also the psychological set of the consulting room, where patients may believe that doctors expect to hear physical rather than psychological complaints. When psychological distress is presented as somatic symptoms, general practitioners often miss the primary diagnosis, as we shall see shortly. In this way, somatization of distress is a common cause of hidden psychiatric morbidity, and goes some way to account for that group who are ill, but whom doctors fail to recognize. We shall return to this issue later in the chapter.

Some patients with psychiatric disorder may have a simultaneous medical condition. The psychiatric state may be secondary, as the co-occurrence of influenza and acute psychosis or the 'emotionally hyperaesthetic infirmities', first described by Bonhoeffer, the psychiatrist father of the theologian (see Jaspers 1962, p. 476). The physical and mental disorders may be independent. Sometimes it is conceivable that they have a common aetiology from a third set of variables. Indeed, there is strong evidence that a subgroup exists in the population who have more physical and psychiatric morbidity than would be expected by chance. This was first suggested by Hinkle and Wolff (1957*a*) and later developed by Taylor and Chave (1964), Shepherd *et al.* (1966), Kreitman *et al.* (1966), and Eastwood (1975). But even when a medical disorder is present, a well-trained doctor should usually be able to identify a co-existing psychiatric illness in its own right, particularly when an association between the two has been established.

PSYCHIATRIC MORBIDITY RECOGNIZED BY GENERAL PRACTITIONERS

This area appears in Fig. 6.1 as circle C. We have noted that some persons are so recognized, but psychiatrists would not see them as cases of psychiatric disorder. They may have eccentricities of behaviour or difficulties in relationships, but they are not mentally ill. It is more important, though, to focus on the remainder of circle C and to consider how more of it might be brought to include those who do have psychiatric symptoms but are not recognized. Goldberg and Blackwell (1970) have called this the *hidden psychiatric morbidity*.

The early exploratory work here was conducted by Kessel (1960), who used the term 'conspicuous psychiatric morbidity'. He defined this as 'attendance during the survey year for one or more illnesses in which an important psychiatric component had been detected by the general practitioner'. In this way, conspicuous psychiatric morbidity is that part which is recognized by general practitioners, the remainder being hidden. Kessel saw three modes by which conspicuous psychiatric morbidity could present: explicit complaints of a psychological nature, such as of anxiety, depression or irritability; somatic complaints not explainable by physical illness, such as palpitations; and an abnormal reaction to a physical disorder. Kessel found that as many as 9 per cent of consulters had such morbidity. Personality defects were not included in this estimate. We would now look upon 9 per cent as far too low a figure. In an important study of 14 general practitioners in London, Shepherd *et al.* (1966, 1981) found a nine-fold variation in the amount of morbidity recognized by them. Although this may be due to people selecting their doctor for his or her receptiveness to psychological complaints, it is more likely that it is the doctors themselves who vary in their readiness or ability to elicit and then recognize psychiatric symptoms. In Mannheim, Germany, B. Cooper (1981) surveyed 1026 adults consulting general practitioners in 13 practices, using the Clinical Interview Schedule (Goldberg *et al.* 1970). He found a case rate of 33 per cent. The rates of psychiatric illness reported by the general practitioners were due more to differing perceptions and diagnostic habits than to real differences in frequency. It is clearly a matter of central importance to understand what causes some psychiatric morbidity to remain unrecognized by general practitioners.

An illustrative study of psychiatric morbidity in general practice

A study of general practices in Manchester gives a good illustration of how morbidity presents, and throws some light on this matter (Bridges and Goldberg 1985). In 13 general practices, nearly 500 persons attending their general practitioners were screened using the General Health Questionnaire (GHQ) (see below). Of 500 individuals having a consultation for any complaint for which there had been no previous attendance with any doctor in the previous 12 months, *one-*

third had psychological symptoms justifying a diagnosis on DSM–III criteria. Two-thirds of these had such a diagnosis *and* a physical disorder. Less than 10 per cent of all the inceptions had only a psychiatric condition. Over half the new consultations were for entirely physical conditions. As few as 17 per cent of the inceptions with a DSM–III diagnosis had *only psychological symptoms*. This is a very striking observation.

Bridges and Goldberg paid particular attention to the presentation of somatic symptoms. They found that over half the patients with a diagnosable psychiatric illness satisfied their criteria for somatization: that the patient had sought help for somatic symptoms of psychiatric illness and did not present psychological symptoms; that the patient attributed the somatic symptoms to a physical illness; that their symptoms justified a diagnosis of a psychiatric disorder by a research psychiatrist at interview; and that treatment of the psychiatric disorder would cause the somatic symptoms to disappear, or revert to their level prior to the episode of psychiatric disorder. A finding of much significance for improving services then emerged. When patients had only psychological symptoms in their psychiatric disorder, 95 per cent were correctly recognized by their family doctor. But when somatization occurred, only half of these cases were correctly recognized. Among the remaining patients with 'hidden psychiatric morbidity', nearly all had a co-existing physical illness. It seems that physical symptoms distract the doctor, so that other aspects of the patient's emotional and social condition tend to be neglected.

THE REDUCTION OF HIDDEN PSYCHIATRIC MORBIDITY

The main reasons for the existence of this group have been reviewed in detail by Sanson-Fisher and Hennrikus (1988). Jencks (1985) has examined it in a United States context. The term 'recognition' implies a dichotomous state: that the distress, symptoms, or disorders are or are not seen to exist by the doctor or other primary care worker. But there are, in fact, some dimensional qualities about this, implying that several levels of recognition exist: for example, the doctor may not record the presence of a psychiatric state in his notes, but may nevertheless prescribe a psychotropic drug, or spend some time in counselling the patient. Where the symptoms are indeed conspicuous and are recognized by the doctor to be quite substantial, there is much to suggest that the classificatory systems presently available are unsuited to the syndromes which present in primary care. These classifications were, after all, developed in psychiatric hospitals and clinics. The consequence may be that many general practitioners do actually recognize that psychological distress is present, but have no appropriate psychiatric category in which to place it.

An important advance has recently been made by Davenport *et al.* (1987) into why psychiatric disorders are sometimes missed during medical consultations. They examined videotapes of interviews by general practitioners, half of whom were known to be highly competent at recognizing psychiatric disorders in their practice; and half of whom were known to be poor at so doing. The authors rated the verbal, vocal, postural, and body movement cues shown by patients during these interviews. The striking finding was that patients with psychiatric disorders showed many fewer cues of their mental state when being interviewed by the less able doctors. The latter actively suppressed the cues of psychological distress in their patients. By contrast, the more able doctors allowed their patients to express more verbal and vocal cues. This study carried important implications for the training of doctors, particularly general practitioners and physicians.

SCREENING IN PRIMARY CARE

When a situation emerges in which it is desirable to identify cases of a disorder, and it is thought that some are being missed or not coming spontaneously to recognition, a *screening* procedure can be introduced. This usually involves a relatively brief test, administered at the initiation of the screening agency, not the persons being tested, as Sackett and Holland (1975) pointed out. In screening for psychiatric disorders, a major contribution has been made by Goldberg (1972, 1985) with the development of the General Health Questionnaire or GHQ. This instrument was developed to detect probable cases in a general practice setting. It has frequently been used in many studies and in many countries specifically to identify the 'hidden psychiatric morbidity'. In this way, it is performing expressly as a screening instrument, for which the criterion for deciding if a person is indeed a case is usually a standardized psychiatric interview. Although much of the work has been conducted in general practices, the methods are just as applicable to general medical patients (Goldberg 1985). The best source of information on this instrument is the user's guide by Goldberg and Williams (1988).

Williams (1986) has reviewed the place of screening in primary care. He notes that only two studies have tried to assess the outcome of screening on treatment by the general practitioner. Johnstone and Goldberg (1976) found no beneficial effect for mild cases, but a profound improvement in severe ones. That is, the general practitioners made good use of the information about severe cases they had not independently recognized by themselves. In a second study (Hoeper *et al.* 1984), it appears that the general practitioner did not make use of the information, for reasons which are unclear. Williams (1986) has drawn together evidence for the following conclusions about screening: it is not justifiable to screen general populations; but it is justifiable to undertake case-finding of psychiatric morbidity in general practice, including hidden morbidity. He draws attention to the need to obtain cost–benefit data on this procedure.

TRAINING GENERAL PRACTITIONERS

Goldberg *et al.* (1980) have gone on to develop a training programme which demonstrably improves general practitioners' recognition of psychiatric illness. Such an intervention programme is an illustration of the application of epidemiological knowledge to achieve better patient care: research had shown unequivocally that a need existed for more efficient recognition of morbidity by general practitioners; a training exercise was designed; and substantial improvements were achieved. The training course has now been evaluated, with highly favourable results (Gask *et al.* 1987, 1988).

The training programme used by Goldberg and his colleagues has two components. First, the baseline performance of trainees is assessed. This can be done by determining their sensitivity in case-detection (the number of cases they recognize amongst all those identified as psychiatric cases by the GHQ or by a clinical interview). It is very desirable in addition to have some qualitative assessment of their attitudes and knowledge about psychiatric symptoms, and of their behaviour and interview style. The second part is the training itself, to be undertaken in small groups or individually, with a psychiatrist who himself has a close familiarity with psychological complaints in general practice. Videotapes of both teacher and trainee are very helpful, with excerpts being used to identify both undesirable behaviours and those which may need to be acquired.

Goldberg and Huxley (1980, p. 136) advocate several components for the training exercise. There should be close attention to the first few minutes of the interview, with both parties sitting comfortably, eye contact ensured, and an open-ended initial enquiry from the doctor. He should then have the patient clarify the initial complaint, being alert to its possibly psychological nature. The interview itself should be controlled: general practitioners are usually under considerable time constraints, but it is nevertheless possible to obtain clinically useful information in a brief period. They are then taught the range of questions which should be asked about general psychological functioning, anxiety symptoms, and depression, working up a hierarchy of severity according to the responses obtained. Having established what symptoms are present, whether these be mainly psychological or somatic manifestations of anxiety or depression, the general practitioner should move on to explore the family and interpersonal context of the patient's current life. This immediate social environment is invariably relevant, either for the origin of the symptoms or the setting in which treatment is to take place.

Having succeeded in enabling general practitioners to have such skills in recognizing psychiatric disorders in their social context, the exercise would be to little avail if they were not also able to undertake appropriate management. They are in an advantageous position to do this, and the appropriate training deserves to be vigorously promoted. This is in the interests of better patient care, the relief of unnecessary suffering for individuals and families and, in many instances, the economic and personal benefits of avoiding needless special investigations.

Algorithms and flow charts to assist management A useful adjunct to face-to-face training is the use of algorithms for the management of individual patients. This may be particularly relevant for the training of non-medical health workers in developing countries. Essex and Gosling (1983) have described a flexible system which has been shown to be both well-accepted and effective.

SOME STUDIES OF PRIMARY CARE

A study of considerable significance for primary care and social psychiatry was initiated and co-ordinated by the World Health Organization, using a paradigm with some similarities to the work by Goldberg (Sartorius and Harding, 1983; Harding *et al.* 1983*a*; Murthy and Wig 1983). The focus was on low-cost methods for providing basic mental health care in developing countries, involving workers already in primary health care facilities. The fieldwork was conducted principally at four sites: a crowded, poor *barrio* near Cali, Colombia; a rural area in Haryana, India; an agricultural zone near Khartoum, Sudan; and a densely populated area in Manila, the Philippines. The essence of the design was (1) to construct, then apply, a simple screening instrument (the Self Reporting Questionnaire) to consecutive attenders; (2) to give the Present State Examination to possible cases; and (3) to compare the morbidity so identified with the cases recognized by workers in the primary care centre. This part of the study confirmed that primary health workers were recognizing only a minority of cases.

The study then moved on to its intervention stage (Harding *et al.* 1983*a*, *b*). In an initial assessment of technical knowledge and attitudes of health workers, Ignacio *et al.* (1983) were able to clarify where deficiencies lay. Staff did not know how to look for psychiatric problems, they had only limited knowledge about psychotropic drugs, and they were unable to contribute personally to the management of cases. Based on this information, the World Health Organization team constructed simple training programmes with a common core, but focusing on particular conditions selected by each site as priorities in its region. These training programmes were demonstrated to be effective in increasing the ability of health workers to recognize mental disorders. For mental disorders in children, the World Health Organization collaborative study was able to demonstrate similar benefits to care through improved case-finding by staff (Giel *et al.* 1981, 1988).

A by-product of this study which is of wider relevance is that interest and attitudes towards mental disorders were substantially improved in primary care staff; and both they and others in the community, including health administrators, spontaneously became more involved in mental health issues. How persistent this change has proved remains to be determined.

Data from the West London Survey with a direct bearing on general practice have been constructively analysed by Williams *et al.* (1986*a*). A survey of West London had been undertaken earlier to investigate, *inter alia*, the effects on health of aircraft noise from Heathrow. Williams and his colleagues showed how it is possible to extract much additional information on other topics by secondary analysis of the data. Such methods are particularly important when large-scale surveys are so costly. They found that minor psychiatric disorder doubled the probability of contact with general practice, and that the principal factors influencing consulting were health-related variables, together with important interaction effects between these and sociodemographic variables.

In South Verona, Tansella *et al.* (1986) made creative use of the Psychiatric Case Register (for mental health services in the region) and a drug prescription monitoring system operating for general practitioners in the very same population. They found that patient contact for affective disorders at the general practitioner level was approximately 10 times greater than at the level of psychiatric out-patients; and the latter was in turn about ten times greater than at the in-patient level.

Classification of psychiatric disorders in primary care

We have noted that the psychiatric states which present in primary care do not fit comfortably into the established classification systems, either ICD–9 or DSM–III. This is an important issue, both scientifically and for health care.

In general practice, psychological or psychiatric morbidity which presents in that setting may differ from hospital-based syndromes in three respects: morbidity in primary care will include less severe states (i.e. with a lower Index of Definition on the PSE); the symptoms often are more fleeting as both Mann *et al.* (1981) and Kessler *et al.* (1985) have now shown; and there could be important differences in the actual array of symptoms, so that the composition of the syndromes may be different. Goldberg (1982) has proposed the following classification on the basis of his experience with morbidity in general practice: (1) major psychiatric illnesses, such as psychoses and severe depressions: (2) psychological distress not requiring specific intervention, but rather a short discussion of current problems: and (3) psychological distress requiring intervention. The latter is a large group. Goldberg further recommends a tri-axial classification in which the first is psychiatric, the second is for physical disorders or symptoms, and the third is for social dysfunction. He points out that the presence of a physical disorder has been shown to make it very much *less* likely that a general practitioner will recognize the co-existent presence of psychological distress. Having both the first and second axes would help to overcome this. Social dysfunction deserves much more explicit recognition. Too little is known about its relationship to impairment on the first two axes, particularly when both psychological and physical symptoms are present together. Although Goldberg's triaxial system is intended for research purposes and was not proposed for routine use, its practical relevance is evident. Furthermore, the patient may not be the only one with social dysfunction, in that the illness may have appreciable effects on the social performance of others in the family (Giel *et al.* 1983). (See also Chapter 5, p. 113 *et seq.*).

SOCIAL WORK AND PSYCHIATRIC CARE

The presence of a significant social component is now acknowledged in all forms of psychiatric disorder, at all ages and in all sections of the community. It is therefore logical that a comprehensive system of mental health care should include attention to both the social origins and the consequences of morbidity. Such effort may also hold the promise of being therapeutic, by shortening the episode and reducing its undesirable social sequelae. This view certainly seems to make good sense for the management of psychiatric disorders, both in primary health care and psychiatric services.

These views have contributed to the overall development of social work as a highly trained profession, and to its playing a key role in services for the mentally ill, as well as its place in general medical services and social welfare. In recent years, there have been a number of important studies in the United Kingdom, Europe, and North America to determine what effects are demonstrable from social work intervention and what groups of patients or clients benefit.

The evidence has not been uniformly encouraging. In the United States, Mullen and Dumpson (1972) reported in their review that researchers 'were rarely able to conclude that a program had even modest success in achieving its major goals'. In 1975, B. Cooper *et al.* reported that in the care of persons with chronic neurotic illnesses, those to whom they randomly allocated social work care, in addition to treatment by their general practitioner, had better social adjustment at the end of the trial. This was unlikely to be due to something specific about social work, but possibly attributable to more time being spent in discussing current troubles than the general practitioner was able to provide. Gibbons *et al.* (1978) randomly assigned social work care to 400 parasuicide patients. There was no difference between the two groups in the principal outcome variable, which was the frequency of subsequent acts of self-poisoning. But the social work group showed an improvement in the way they viewed their problems. In a much discussed trial of social work intervention for truanting in Leeds, Berg *et al.* (1978) found that the experimental group subsequently had *more* truanting and *more* delinquent acts than the control group of young persons.

In an earnest book, *Can social work survive?*, Brewer and Lait (1980) examined evidence for the effectiveness of social work in all sectors of care, but particularly in relation to health services. These authors suggested that social workers are usually closely wedded to their beliefs about the style of their work and are resistant to changes to that style in the face of evidence. The strongly psychodynamic tradition underlying the general philosophy of social work may have contributed to this in some centres.

More recent work from the General Practice Research Unit in London has done much to clarify the relationship between general practice and social work in the care of the mentally ill. For patients with chronic neuroses, B. Cooper *et al.* (1975) conducted a controlled trial of attaching a social worker to a group practice in London. They found that the experimental service conferred some benefit to the patients. Corney (1982) compared the outcome in depressed women who were randomly assigned care by a social worker in addition to routine care by their general practitioners. This study provided a description of what care was actually given by the social workers. They used 'sustaining' techniques, trying to determine why the patient was depressed, and offering support. They gave help in understanding the simple dynamics of the situation. Behavioural techniques were also used, through setting tasks for the depressed woman to get through in the day, and establishing a contact between her and her spouse or boyfriend to increase their co-operation. The social workers also offered practical help. Only one subgroup was found to benefit: those who had been depressed for a long time and who had a poor relationship with the husband or boyfriend. This finding fits well with the findings of Brown and his colleagues on vulnerability factors in depressed women (Brown and Harris 1978; Harris *et al.* 1987; Harris, (1988). Corney (1984) has since looked at the adequacy of communication between general practitioners and social workers caring for the same patients. She found that the contacts were very limited.

What seems to be happening is that social work in common with other caring activities, such as psychotherapy, has begun to undergo critical assessment. Such evaluation is helping to clarify how this highly motivated professional resource can be most effectively engaged in managing the social distress which is so abundant in most urban communities. There can indeed be difficulties between social workers and medical or other staff. It seems usually to be of an ethological nature, to do with dominance hierarchies and professional or intellectual territory. The comprehensive care of the mentally ill and their families cannot readily be achieved by medical personnel alone. As well as social workers, it is now well-known that community psychiatric nurses, health visitors, and psychologists are making major contributions. In the context of community care, Clare and Corney (1982) therefore rightly assert that: 'The issue is not whether social workers and general practitioners should collaborate in providing a truly integrated system of health and social care, but rather whether they can afford not to do so'. A succinct review of these issues has been set out by Corney (1985). If this area of applied social psychiatry is to contribute to health care in the next century, some effort will be needed to promote mutual esteem among the professionals involved; and to demonstrate what social interventions are useful and practicable.

CLINICAL PSYCHOLOGY AND PRIMARY CARE

A matter which is of high importance for the future of psychiatry is the role of the clinical psychologist. Some of the issues have been set out in the volume edited by McPherson and Sutton (1981). Here we are concerned with the contribution of the clinical psychologist to primary care. Succinct reviews, with an examination of the principal problems, have been written by Spector (1984) and by Marteau and Johnston (1987). Other useful accounts of the situation in Britain are by Broadhurst (1972) and Clark (1979), and Rappaport (1977) has described the development of community psychology in the United States.

From the 1960s, clinical psychologists began to be involved in patient care in the community, mainly through general practices and community clinics. In a number of countries, University Departments of Psychology began to establish links with their local general practices, conscious of the contribution they might make to the abundant psychosocial disorder which presents there; and aware of the research opportunities such settings can afford. Primary care staff, including general practitioners, do not see psychiatrists as necessarily the first professional group to engage in helping their clientele. Clinical psychologists are correctly perceived as another likely source of help.

The service contribution by clinical psychologists has usually been in direct therapeutic activities, mostly one-to-one with patients. McPherson (1981) and Spector (1984), among many others, have pointed to the other contributions which could also be made in preventive, educational, and research activities. Evaluation of therapeutic work has been carried out, as by Earll and Kincey (1982) in Britain, and Brodaty and Andrews (1983) in Australia. No significant differences were found in the outcome between general practitioner- and psychologist-treated cases of minor psychiatric disorder. As for the views of UK general practitioners on the usefulness of clinical psychologists, Eastman and McPherson (1982) found they rated them eighth out of 10 professions, equal with psychiatrists. Clearly, there is much mutual education required, and this is probably necessary before clinical psychologists can make progress in the other areas of prevention, education of patients and research.

Spector (1984) draws attention to an area of difficulty which is the same as that encountered by social work in primary care. This is a different perception of how primary care should be organized. Some see it as a generalist *service* in which several professions collaborate to one end; others see it as a service provided by a *generalist* (the general practitioner) who draws on the expertise of locally based specialists (e.g. surgeons, paediatricians, social workers, dieticians, and other professionals). These issues of an ethological nature, concerning dominance hierarchies and territories, are likely to present serious impediments for a long time to come. Yet true collaboration *can* be achieved when there is well-founded mutual respect, a common sense of commitment, well-defined areas of professional competence, and a spirit of enquiry.

CONCLUSIONS AND FUTURE PROSPECTS

There is now a great deal of useful information about mental disorders in primary care. The advances in knowledge over only two decades have been impressive, although they have come from only a handful of researchers. The field remains a fertile one for further work, and carries the dual attraction of being manifestly useful for patient care and, at the same time, raising some fundamental issues in social and clinical psychiatry, and in health economics.

One central question remains unanswered, yet of the greatest relevance for progress in the immediate future. Shepherd (1987) has pointed to the unanimous view that general medical and mental health services should be more closely integrated; yet governments do not show by their behaviour that they wish to overcome the main impediments to this. And there has to be doubt that the majority of general practitioners are both able and willing to undertake a central role in the management of patients with psychiatric disorders.

In the light of these uncertainties, it is now necessary to take stock of where social psychiatry and epidemiology stand in this field, both for further useful enquiry and for intervention strategies. There has been much advance in knowledge, but much of that knowledge, and its implications for practice and policy, now needs to be applied at national levels. In an agenda for the immediate future, a prominent item is the recognition and management of psychiatric disorders in special groups, such as the elderly or adolescents. In this, as in the role of general practitioners for all sectors of the population, public expectations of their performance may prove to be a constructive driving force for greater competence. This will need much activity by the institutions concerned; and close collaboration between general practitioners, the research community, and administrators.

7

Social treatments and preventive strategies

Introduction; social treatments for childhood disorders; neuroses; affective disorders; schizophrenia; expressed emotion: the original observation, measurement, findings in schizophrenia, characteristics in relatives, in other disorders, intervention programmes, conclusions. Social treatments of dementia; alcohol and drug dependency; knowledge available for prevention in psychiatry: the World Health Organization recommendations.

INTRODUCTION

At the same time that social psychiatry has pursued clues to aetiology and factors which influence outcome, it has also made many major contributions to the treatment and after-care of mental disorders; and in a few instances, it has been able to point the way to strategies for prevention. We shall use the matrix in Table 3.2 as a framework for examining both issues (see p. 34).

Two distinct principles can be discerned in social psychiatric treatments. In the first category, there are efforts to alter the environment around the individual, in the belief that a change in the behaviour of others, or in the level of social stimulation, will diminish symptoms. We shall see this exemplified below for childhood disorders, schizophrenia and dementia. The focus of attention is on the quality of the immediate social environment, the expectation being that a change will benefit the patient's mental state. To achieve this, patients have exposure to certain environments prescribed as part of their treatment plan. Efforts are directed towards altering the social environment, particularly in the way that the family and others behave towards the patient. In the second category, patients can be taught how to handle or cope with anticipated situations which may present difficulties, commonly using some form of practice or rehearsal to equip themselves with a protective behaviour, which can then be invoked when needed. Here the focus of attention is quite different from the previous category: there is no attempt to change the environment or the person's exposure to different experiences.

Instead, attention is directed at having the patient become more socially skilled and better able to respond to those stressor experiences which can be expected to impinge on him from his social environment. Of all such social treatments, the most developed and the most widely practiced is psychotherapy. The social components of this, common to all the psychotherapies and traditional healing practices, have been examined by Jerome Frank in his outstanding contribution to our understanding of this field. Anyone who pretends an interest in social psychiatry will be enriched by reading *Persuasion and healing* (Frank 1973), and some of his seminal papers (Frank 1974, 1977, 1986). Essential social ingredients for successful psychotherapy are that the sufferer wants relief from his demoralization, that he seeks help from a person designated as having the capability to heal, and that the two persons have a shared system of beliefs about the nature and origin of the problem.

CHILDHOOD DISORDERS

There is now a sizeable literature on the social components of treating neurotic and conduct disorders, mental retardation, and childhood psychoses. These have been comprehensively detailed in a major work by Rutter and Hersov (1985). Emphasis tends to be on the two categories of social treatment mentioned above. In neurotic and conduct disorders, the key to management is very largely to work with the parents, so that their responses may be altered in a way which, in time, will bring about changes in the child's behaviour. Exposure to well-specified environments is also useful in reducing anxiety symptoms, lessening withdrawal, and controlling behaviour disorders. This is in fact the essence of special schooling, the principles of play therapy and treatment sessions in children's clinics. It is a field which offers rich opportunities for evaluation research.

Family therapy

A social treatment of particular use for children is family therapy. Here there is now a number of useful introductions and expositions of the principles, giving the newcomer a helpful cognitive map to serve as a guide (Ackerman 1966; Haley 1971). The present writer has found the chapter by Bentovim (1986) a clearly written account. Bentovim proposes that a successfully functioning family should include the following: a setting in which each can fulfil his potential; a model for socialization which can be transferred to the world outside; models in the parents for sexual identity; and boundaries demarcating parent and children whereby the latter accept and can respect the leadership role of the parents. A family is considered to be made up of several subsystems, each bound by a set of rules.

In family therapy, one approach aims at modifying the family structure so that subsystems form which can work in harmony. This is achieved by bringing about changes in communication. Bentovim gives as an example encouraging a mother to set aside regular times to talk with her teenage daughter, where such communication was not previously taking place. This approach is along the lines developed by Minuchin (1974, 1984).

Another approach which depends on improving communication is called strategic therapy (Haley 1971, 1977). Here, emphasis is placed on the setting of well-specified goals closely related to the presenting problem. The family therapist is active in calling for changes in the way members relate. Bentovim points out that this style of family therapy deals only with the present and does not attempt to generate members' self-understanding. A third type of family therapy is behavioural, based on the principles of learning theory, whereby a change of behaviour by one member is reinforced by reciprocal changes in others.

The amount of information available on the effectiveness of social interventions with children and young persons, including family therapy, remains seriously deficient, and is far from commensurate with the effort currently invested in such treatment by highly trained and professionally committed personnel. But as Bloch and Crouch (1985) have shown in their volume on group psychotherapy, empirical research can now be improved because methodologies have been developed to a level where both the design and measurement are now adequate for the task.

NEUROSES

Both categories of social treatment can be applied to adults with neurotic disorders. Changes in the behaviour of others is often highly relevant, because the existing pattern may be maintaining the patient's symptoms through reinforcement. These symptoms may, in the first instance, be a maladaptive response to a domestic environment which is seriously amiss. This is commonly the background to neurotic depression, parasuicide, or somatic symptoms, as in the setting of an unhealthy marriage. The person with the symptoms may be found to be conspicuously deficient in care and concern from the spouse or other family members, but attempts to correct this may result in engaging in care-eliciting behaviour which is considered socially deviant (Henderson 1974). The symptoms or behaviour can have a profound effect on others. Such states, particularly those with somatic symptoms of psychological origin, are probably very common in general practice and psychiatric out-patient clinics (Bridges and Goldberg, 1985). Once the interpersonal context is uncovered, it provides a clear guide to social treatment. The agenda thereby generated is a rich one for both individual and conjoint therapy. In the conduct of this, it is very important to obtain detailed information from both parties; and on that basis to work towards a closer relationship, in which mutual requirements can be met more satisfactorily. Where the behaviour of others, including family members, has little to do with the onset of a neurotic disorder or its maintenance, it is invariably useful to counsel the spouse about the nature of the disorder and how he or she should respond to the patient in the course of daily life. Such attention to spouses and other family members tends to be often neglected.

In the category of social treatment of neurosis and personality disorders, it is appropriate to place group psychotherapy, and, in addition, the even more complex social processes which characterize a therapeutic community. Such principles are now in wide use, for example in the rehabilitation of drug dependent persons. The social and psychological factors in group psychotherapy have been thoroughly examined by Bloch and Crouch (1985) in their useful review.

In agoraphobia and social phobias, socially-oriented behaviour therapy, through graded exposure to feared social situations, is now an established strategy in treatment. It is undoubtedly effective, and *in vivo* exposure seems to be more effective than the imagined presentation of the stimulus. For a comprehensive account of the theory and practice of behavioural psychotherapy, the reader is referred to the work of Marks (1969, 1981). As a social component of treatment programmes for anxiety disorders, it is useful to have the patients meet together to discuss their difficulties and encourage each other in progress. This has a beneficial effect for several reasons: patients consistently report that it is helpful to learn they are not unique in their affliction; there is a group effect in having a shared goal; and participation in speaking in front of others is helpful for those with specific social fears and low self-confidence.

AFFECTIVE DISORDERS

The contribution of social methods in the treatment of affective disorders comes mainly from the second method listed above: patients may benefit from training in how to handle their social environment more effectively. This is the essence of cognitive therapy for depression, where changes are sought in the way the external world is perceived and interpreted. An account of the principles and practice of cognitive therapy is set out in the volumes by Beck (1976) and Beck *et al.* (1979), and in a subsequent paper by Seligman (1981). An overview of cognitive theories of depression is to be found in Power (1987). Some activity in the first category of intervention can also be relevant: it is usually very helpful to determine how other family members have responded to the patient's depressive symptoms.

SCHIZOPHRENIA

More than in any other diagnostic group, social methods have made a substantial contribution to the management of schizophrenia. This is attributable to the research effort and initiative of some pioneers in social psychiatric care. The earliest efforts were in the rehabilitation of schizophrenics into life outside hospital. An account of the issues involved can be found in Wing and Brown (1970) and Wing (1978*a*). The social treatments developed for schizophrenia fell into two related categories: strategies for rehabilitation towards more normal patterns of living; and the reduction of undesirable components in interpersonal transactions, including what has come to be known as 'expressed emotion'. We shall deal with each in turn.

In 1961, Wing and Freudenberg reported that severely ill chronic schizophrenic patients improved when their level of social stimulation in hospital was experimentally increased. This finding was based on the detailed study of 22 patients. Their supervision in a hospital workshop was conducted at two levels: passive, with minimal social interaction being given by the nursing staff; and active, where staff gave praise and encouragement, set clear goals, but desisted if patients showed irritation. The output of the patients on a simple task was strikingly improved by 'active' supervision. The authors found no change in the patient's mental state or ward behaviour.

In the same year, Wing and Brown (1961) reported a study contrasting three mental hospitals which differed in their social conditions and administrative policies. They found a consistent pattern: at the hospital where there had been considerable reforms, clinical disturbance of the patients was least. Wing and Brown gave due consideration to selection effects as an explanation for this gradient, but were able to conclude that social conditions in mental hospitals do influence the mental state of schizophrenic patients. It is now clear that the social environment in which patients are treated for chronic mental disorders has a marked influence on their social adjustment and performance in daily living.

These findings provided much encouragement for the development of effective, rationally based programmes for the treatment of the severely mentally ill. It was a new area of research, which opened the way to treatments complementary to medication, the combination of both pharmacological and social treatment proving powerful. Principles of rehabilitation began to be articulated, based on the needs of patients facing the world outside hospital. In an influential paper, Wing (1966) described the changes in social conditions and self-confidence which took place in a group of 12 persons passing through an Industrial Rehabilitation Unit. He found that a majority improved in self-confidence and were able to find outside employment. Significantly, their initial attitude to their difficulties was a strong predictor of outcome.

The value of such studies has been far-reaching. They have influenced administrative policy in the provision of services for the mentally ill. They have shown that it is demonstrably worthwhile to develop the residual capacities of severely disabled patients. And they have established a tradition of scientific activity in this part of psychiatry and public health which deals with chronic disorders. For a particularly good account of the principles and practice of social treatments in psychiatry, including rehabilitation, the chapter by Bennett (1978) is strongly recommended. In his volume *Reasoning about madness*, Wing (1978*b*) has included a chapter which describes the development of services for the mentally ill, how these have differed in Britain, the United States, and the Soviet Union, and what the strengths and weaknesses are in current practices, particularly in relation to psychosis.

EXPRESSED EMOTION

How this area of social psychiatry has evolved is worth the reader's close attention. It is very interesting to follow through the sequence of developments, and there is much to be learned from noting the principles at work. The study of expressed emotion began as a largely unexpected research finding which has been steadily developed over nearly three decades to become one of the more notable successes in psychiatric care. The significance of this body of research for the well-being of many thousands of psychiatric patients must be considerable. The subject will clearly lend itself in the future to a detailed historical review.

A small group of social scientists and clinicians made an unexpected finding about social factors in the outcome for discharged schizophrenic patients; they were alert to it and followed it up. Others have subsequently looked in greater detail at the patients' immediate social environment; they have identified some of the pathogenic elements fairly specifically, then derived an intervention which benefits patients and their families. It may be added that, in addition, a rich seam has been opened up on fundamental issues concerning social behaviour, in health and in the context of mental illness. Here is a subject matter for continuing research relevant to patient care and to an understanding of human interaction. A reasonable expectation is that expressed emotion will come to have relevance outside the immediate clinical areas of schizophrenia and depression. It may lead to knowledge for prevention in other domains, such as parental style in raising children, and enhancement of well-being in families. The present state of knowledge about expressed emotion has been thoroughly reviewed by Hooley (1986), following the earlier review by Kuipers (1979). The definitive source is the book by Leff and Vaughn (1985).

The original observation

In 1958, Brown, Carstairs, and Topping had been studying schizophrenic patients at the Maudsley Hospital, London, in terms of how they fared after discharge from in-patient care. They noted that patients who returned to live in lodgings or with siblings had a lower relapse rate than those who went to live with parents or spouses. It was also noted that patients who spent more time in direct contact with relatives had a higher relapse rate (Brown *et al.* 1962; Wing *et al.*

1964). They then used a prospective design in which they measured 'emotion expressed', 'hostility', and 'dominance' in both the patients and their relatives. They found that relapse was higher in families with high hostility or expressed emotion (EE). This led them to construct and then refine an instrument for measuring EE, called the Camberwell Family Interview (Brown and Rutter 1966; Rutter and Brown 1966), which takes 3–4 hours to administer. Vaughn and Leff (1976) later developed a shortened version.

Measurement of expressed emotion

The observation that interpersonal transactions and the emotional climate of the home could influence relapse in schizophrenia has been the basis for most of the subsequent research. A central role in this has been played by the family interview. It is administered to key relatives and should be audiotaped for subsequent ratings and analysis. The respondent is asked about the onset of the illness and events in the home during the three months before the patient's entry to care, and about his or her feeling towards the patient and the disorder. The ratings of EE are made from the relative's responses. Five distinct ratings are made: criticism, hostility, emotional over-involvement, warmth, and positive remarks. Most attention has so far been paid to the first three of these, because only they appear to be predictors of relapse, although the other two are of continuing interest as possible modifying factors.

Criticism is based on the content of remarks, and on voice–tone changes. Hostility is a different construct, because it refers not to remarks about specific behaviours, but to general feelings and attitudes to the patient as a person. Emotional over-involvement is akin to the constructs of excessive concern and protection in parental style (see p. 73). It refers to an excessive emotional response by the relative to the patient's illness and its implications.

Findings on schizophrenia

A strong association has consistently been found between high levels of criticism and/or emotional over-involvement on the one hand, and subsequent relapse. This work has since been replicated with close attention to method by Vaughn and her colleagues (Vaughn and Leff, 1976; Vaughn *et al.* 1982). The measures are made before the patient's discharge, and the follow-up period has been nine months to one year. Hooley (1986) has pointed out that the definition of relapse is not confounded by antagonistic attitudes to the patient, which might also lead to his or her admission, thereby producing a spurious association. There are now reports that the association holds in cultures other than European. It has been confirmed twice in Los Angeles (Vaughn *et al.* 1984; Karno *et al.* 1987) and in Chandigarh (Leff *et al.* 1987; Wig *et al.* 1987*a*, *b*). In the Chandigarh study, first-contact schizophrenic patients had a significantly better outcome than a London sample. The proportion of relatives with high expressed emotion was also much lower, leading Leff and his colleagues to conclude that this was in large part the reason for the more favourable outcome for schizophrenia in Chandigarh. As Hooley has perceptively pointed out, studies which do *not* find an association between high EE and subsequent relapse are valuable because they may provide clues about how EE operates. They may also provide more specific information on what type of patient does or does not relapse under high EE.

There is already good evidence that three factors interact with EE. These are the time spent by the patient with high EE relatives, medication, and independent life events. Brown *et al.* (1962) had found in their earlier studies that patients were partly protected from high EE relatives if their time in contact with them was limited. Neuroleptic medication can also provide a partial umbrella against EE. Vaughn and Leff (1976) combined data from both Brown *et al.* (1972) and their own study to show that patients in high EE environments, but who were both on medication and had less than 35 hours per week with the high EE relatives, had a relapse rate of only 15 per cent, which was the same as low EE patients. By contrast, patients with high EE relatives, more than 35 hours contact per week, and no medication, had a relapse rate of 92 per cent. For independent life events, the data suggest that these are particularly associated with relapse in patients from low EE homes (Leff and Vaughn 1980); and that life-events have much less of an impact on patients living in high EE environments.

The latter finding may at first appear puzzling. But a new segment of EE research goes some way to explain it. Efforts to link psychosocial events or attributes with biological measures have been all too rare in psychiatry. Some EE workers, however, have used a psychophysiological measure to try to link social experiences and biological changes, monitoring skin conductance during interviews with a psychiatrist and, later in the session, in the presence of a high

EE relative (Tarrier *et al.* 1979; Sturgeon *et al.* 1981, 1984). The results have not been very consistent, but it does seem that encounters with high EE relatives are more emotionally arousing than with low EE relatives. Sturgeon *et al.* have put forward an attractive hypothesis that the rise in skin conductance which takes place during a relapse in low EE patients is a more transient phenomenon than the larger-sustained rise in those with high EE. They propose that high EE patients are exposed to more chronic environmental stress, so that additional life events understandably have little additional effect. By contrast, life events impinging on low EE patients make for a more acute stress.

What characterizes high and low EE relatives

It would be useful to understand what attributes distinguish the two types of relatives, because this could be applied to treatment and secondary prevention. Surprisingly, EE is not easy to recognize without training. The construct is not obvious to the unprepared observer. Vaughn (1986) and Vaughn and Leff (1981) have undertaken content analyses of critical remarks by relatives, identifying those response styles which distinguish high from low EE persons. These are (1) intrusiveness, often in the form of fussing and persistence in giving unsolicited help; (2) a more dramatic response to the patient's illness by high EE individuals; (3) less inclination to believe the patient is ill; and (4) lower tolerance of the patient's behaviour and his diminished performance. It is not yet known if these are stable attributes like personality traits, if they are relatively recent attributes developed in response to having a sick family member, or if they are situational and person-specific, being directed only at the schizophrenic family member.

EE in other psychiatric disorders

Vaughn and Leff (1976) were the first to show that high EE was also associated with relapse in neurotic depression, and that there is an interaction with life-events (Leff and Vaughn 1980). Indeed, it is improbable that high EE has an effect in the relapse of only schizophrenia. This suggests that the EE hypothesis could be applied in further exploratory studies with other diagnostic groups, such as alcoholism, somatization disorder, anorexia or bulimia nervosa, and anxiety disorders. In this way, the matrix in Table 3.2 leads to several plausible hypotheses worth pursuing (p. 34).

Interventions using the EE model

Intervention studies in EE carry the double attraction of developing a highly promising therapeutic intervention to help families, and of making a powerful contribution towards understanding the direction of causality in the association. For the latter, it could be that the patients in high EE families were more disturbed in the first place and more likely to relapse, leading to a misleading association. Against such an interpretation, Brown *et al.* (1972), Vaughn and Leff (1976) and Vaughn *et al.* (1984) had taken great care in their diagnosis and analyses to avoid this. Leff *et al.* (1982) have now developed an intervention, based on a training package for families with a schizophrenic member. In preliminary trials, its effectiveness is impressive. A manual has been prepared as a guide for relatives seeking self-help (see also Chapter 5, p. 114–15).

Conclusion

As indicated at the beginning of this section, EE research is a good example of how a research finding has been developed and carried through with persistent effort to a stage where it now significantly illuminates part of the disease process, and provides a soundly based, effective intervention for treatment and secondary prevention. Finally, it should be firmly recognized that the EE hypothesis refers to relapse, not to onset, and has not been proposed as a factor in the aetiology of schizophrenia or depression.

DEMENTIA

Social treatments of the dementias of later life fall largely into the first of the categories in the introduction to this chapter. A well-organized and comprehensive review of psychosocial interventions in dementia is by Whitehead (1984). There is good reason to believe that a dreary environment and the premature loss of personal autonomy may serve only to accelerate decline in cognitive functioning. It may also make the addition of depressive symptoms more likely in the early stages. This can take place in the patient's own home as readily as in a nursing home or residential hostel. For example, Langer and Rodin (1976) showed that enhancement of personal responsibility and increase in opportunities to make choices promoted alertness and well-being in elderly residents of a nursing home. Accordingly, those living or working with elderly patients with cognitive impairment or dementia should allow as much personal responsibility and choice as possible. Family members are nearly always helped towards greater tolerance of repeated questioning, wandering, irritability, and other difficult behaviour, if they are assured that these are the products of an illness, and that they are not deliberate on the part of the patient.

Whitehead (1984) lists five categories of psychosocial intervention in dementia: milieu therapy, activity engagement, physical exercise, problem-oriented approaches, and reality orientation. In milieu therapy, the aim is to reinstate ordinary styles of living to an institutional environment. Examples are having small tables for meals, napkins, and attractive table appointments, or arranging seating so that people can more readily interact. Recreational activities can be promoted by making materials very immediately available to persons with dementia. In trials, the effects have consistently been favourable, with a decrease in inactivity and some increase in socialization. Physical activity has been demonstrated to improve cognitive performance in dementia patients in institutional care, although there was no change in ratings of behaviour.

Application of learning theory principles has been assessed for behaviours which cause difficulties. This problem-oriented approach is directed at behaviour such as shouting, poor self-care, or incontinence. It is uncertain at what stage such intervention is best attempted, or whether milieu therapy is more effective. Clearly, in a disorder characterized by impairment of learning new material, there will be considerable limitations.

Where exposure to a special environment is advocated, the social treatment is termed 'reality orientation therapy'. Here, the patient is vigorously exposed to basic information about the setting, date, and day of the week, and the basic social context of his own existence. In senile dementia of Alzheimer type, it is at least conceivable that a stimulating environment, which makes full use of what cognitive resources remain, may slow the deterioration in functional performance, if not the progression of the neuropathological changes. Woods (1979) found reality orientation was effective in improving memory and cognitive performance in elderly persons in residential care. Continued improvement was achieved by Reeve and Ivison (1985) by having continued exposure to reality orientation together with simple modification to the physical environment to provide cues for orientation. Melin and Götestam (1981) also found that minor changes in the environment brought about improvement in the social behaviour of patients with senile dementia. By making recreational activities available in a psychogeriatric unit, and by stimulation to use them in those who did not initiate activities, Jenkins *et al.* (1977) were able to bring about an increased level of engagement in activity. Such studies are a few of the many which now make it clear that psychosocial stimulation, with active involvement of staff, has a beneficial effect on cognitive performance and behaviour. But Whitehead (1984) concludes from her review of 11 studies that the results are inconsistent. In residential settings, these psychosocial treatments for dementia do seem able to improve some aspects of intellectual functioning and to improve behaviour, although there is also evidence for some detrimental effects from reality orientation, enhanced stimulation, and prompted recreational activity. This may be because increasing activity does make all behaviour more probable, including those that are disruptive. It is nevertheless encouraging to see that interest in psychosocial treatments has increased recently, with the promise of further refinements being developed for application both in institutional settings and in the community.

A specific category of social treatment of the elderly with mental disorder is the use of day centres, and respite or shared care. The real value of day centres may lie in providing a brief period of freedom from responsibility for the patient's closest relative, commonly a spouse or daughter. This is explicitly the case in respite or shared care, where the patient is admitted for a brief period to allow his or her family some relief. Day centres may also provide cognitive and social stimulation for persons who are otherwise deprived of this.

ALCOHOL AND DRUG DEPENDENCY

Social treatment and rehabilitation of alcohol or drug-dependent persons is now a major field, which is not reviewed here. There is also the question of social policies which influence the availability of alcohol and access to drugs of dependence. This has now become a field of considerable public health relevance.

For specific modalities of treatment, the social component of Alcoholics Anonymous is quite explicit, as it is for similar organizations for spouses and for drug dependency. In most clinical programmes, it is recognized that a change in the immediate social environment, particularly in the behaviour of others towards the alcoholic or drug addict, may help promote fragile self-esteem. Specific environments have been prescribed, usually to contrast with the urban setting where the alcohol or drug dependency began. In some Scandinavian programmes, emphasis is placed on hard physical exertion, presumably to provide a distraction and to promote a sense of well-being. In social rehabilitation, it seems very reasonable to offer alcoholics and drug addicts opportunities to rehearse how they will cope with situations in which there is a temptation to resume their habit.

KNOWLEDGE AVAILABLE FOR PREVENTION

Prevention in psychiatry sometimes has come to be seen sceptically, even negatively, although such a view is now regarded as seriously mistaken. Here we shall try to establish basic definitions, then select some categories of disorder for consideration. *Primary prevention* brings about reduction of the incidence of a disorder. *Secondary prevention* causes shortening of the duration of a disorder, minimizing the chance of its spread to other persons or reducing the likelihood of the onset of a second, super-added disorder. *Tertiary prevention* refers to measures to limit the disability and handicap which may follow a disorder or the impairment it brings. It will be apparent that some overlap can exist. For example, minimizing the chances of spread to others can be called secondary prevention, but it would also bring about a reduction in fresh incidence, which itself is primary prevention.

Neurosis and affective disorders

No success can yet be claimed in the primary prevention of these, but recent work on parental style (see Chapter 4, p. 73) now points directly to such a possibility. A drop in neurotic and affective disorders in subsequent adult life would be predicted if parents shifted their behaviour, where necessary, to become more caring and less controlling. Demonstration of such an effect would, of course, require a prospective study lasting some decades, with an experimental design. Such an opportunity is unlikely to be available, but the theoretical basis which justifies it is attractive. Jorm (1987) has examined the evidence for trying to reduce neuroticism as a risk factor, using techniques such as rational emotive therapy in high schools or colleges.

Significant contributions to secondary and tertiary prevention are likely to be attributable to the advent of antidepressant medication, and to the availability of both general practitioners and psychiatric services. These are each likely to have made a sizeable contribution to shortening the length of episodes, their recurrence, and their associated disabilities. But formal demonstration of such effects is difficult to obtain for total populations. Recent developments in the cognitive treatment of depression may again hold considerable relevance for secondary and tertiary prevention.

Perhaps one of the greatest challenges in the immediate future is tertiary prevention in the chronic neurotic disorders. A proportion of such patients embark on a life of invalidity, sometimes endorsed by government pensions, or seek compensation in court for an injury which has produced a degree of disability much in excess of the physical changes induced. Reduction in what Pilowsky (1969, 1988) has termed abnormal illness behaviour would indeed be a worthwhile effort in tertiary prevention.

Schizophrenia

The present writer is unaware of any primary preventive measure against schizophrenia which would be practicable. In secondary and tertiary prevention, there is more scope. The work on expressed emotion provides an outstanding example of a demonstrable reduction in relapse rates following intervention (see p. 148). Neuroleptic medication has similarly been shown to be indisputably useful, although not for every patient (Leff and Wing 1971).

In tertiary prevention, the objective is to reduce undesirable consequences which may otherwise become grafted onto the disorder itself. The 'institutional neurosis' described by Barton (1966) was such a state, characterized by loss of initiative and motivation for personal responsibility, a typical posture and gait, and the lack of basic competence in social skills. It typically occurred in long-stay psychotic patients in mental hospitals. Revision of the pattern of care brought about a reduction in these added disabilities. The social breakdown syndrome described by Gruenberg (1974), which is a quite separate entity, is an example *par excellence* of the need for tertiary prevention in the care of the severely mentally ill. This, too, refers to the reduction of disability in social competence (Gruenberg and Kennedy. 1988).

Dementia

Because the dementias are amongst the most threatening disorders of later life, their prevention and early treatment are of great importance, both for families and for national budgets. This subject has been recently reviewed by a World Health Organization Scientific Group on Senile Dementia, in its report *Dementia in later life: Research and action* (WHO 1985*a*). For multi-infarct dementia, it is still unclear if reduction of hypertension will reduce its incidence. Some of the angiopathy may be independent of hypertension. For Alzheimer's disease, including its senile form, there is no primary prevention yet known. In the secondary prevention of the dementias, there are many opportunties. These include:

- the treatment of intercurrent physical illness;
- the treatment of psychotic manifestations;
- the management of behavioural problems with tranquillizers, anti-epileptic medication, where appropriate, and the use of appropriate hypnotics;
- psychological interventions to control behavioural problems;
- counselling and support of families;
- treatment of associated depressive disorder.

As yet, no drug has been shown to arrest or reverse the changes of Alzheimer's disease, although there are some promising developments (e.g. Summers *et al.* 1986). Early detection and screening have been advocated; however, the implications for persons and for services need careful consideration (B. Cooper and Bickel 1984; Henderson and Huppert 1984). Psychological and social interventions have been carried out on persons with dementia in institutional settings, as discussed earlier in this chapter. Interventions with families who look after relatives with dementia has come to be recognized as an important preventive activity (Braithwaite 1987), because these carers are known to have an increased incidence of psychological symptoms. Much can be achieved by counselling and education on strategies to cope with difficult behaviour. Admission of the elderly person to residential care is known to be followed by an immediate improvement in the carer's mental health (Wells and Jorm 1987), although this transition itself may call for sensitive counselling to minimize guilt on the part of a spouse, son or daughter.

THE WORLD HEALTH ORGANIZATION RECOMMENDATIONS ON PREVENTION

In 1985, the World Health Organization prepared a report on the *Prevention of mental, neurological and psychosocial disorders*. This was presented by the Director General to the Thirty-Ninth World Health Assembly (WHO 1985*b*; see also Eisenberg 1987). The report represents a mile-stone in public health. Its architects have considered the whole range of pathology and disorder in the mental, neurological, and psychosocial fields seen from a global perspective, and from the viewpoint of both developed and less developed countries. Entry points for preventive action have then been sought, with the assertion that implementation of a comprehensive programme of prevention *based on methods currently available* could produce a substantial reduction of suffering, of the destruction of human potential, and of the economic loss produced by this large category of disorders. It is envisaged that such a programme would attack both the biological and the social causes which underlie these disorders. A vital element is that, for success, the programme requires national commitment and co-ordinated actions in many social sectors.

The Report sees prevention as having to take place at three levels, which have to be co-ordinated: the health sector, other social sectors, and government policy. Some activities will prevent the occurrence of mental, neurological, and psychosocial disorders (primary prevention); others will minimize chronic disability of impairment or disease. The following is a summary of the recommendations.

1. Preventing the occurrence of morbidity
   - (i) Measures to reduce risk of social and cognitive failure:
     - (a) Enriched day care for children, particularly for families that are unable to provide appropriate stimulation.
     - (b) Enhancing the human environment in long-term care institutions, whether for the young or old, or for the physically or the mentally handicapped.
     - (c) Education for parenthood, where parents lack the relevant skills and have insufficient knowledge of children's needs. This may have to become a responsibility of public education.
     - (d) Introduction of health education in school curricula, to include pre-marital counselling, family life, human sexua-

lity, child development, nutrition, accident prevention, and substance abuse.

(ii) Measures in primary health care and in schools to control substance abuse.

(iii) Measures to reduce the health consequences of acute stress through intervention in primary health care. There is some evidence that counselling of the bereaved or those exposed to other stressor experiences, including divorce, can diminish risk (Raphael 1977, 1983; Bloom *et al.* 1985). Crisis intervention units have been shown to handle effectively a variety of acute mental health problems, and to prevent the development of more chronic difficulties and social disadvantages in the recipients (J. Cooper 1979).

(iv) Measures to prevent iatrogenic damage in primary health care. Here it is argued that health personnel can be trained to recognize psychosocial problems when evaluating new patients. This in turn allows them to recognize symptoms which are expressions of psychological distress and to avoid misuse of psychotropic or other medication. Brief counselling or referral to social or mental health workers can be effective in reducing later morbidity and the frequency of clinic visits. Avoidance of unnecessary hospitalization in children is advocated to avoid the behavioural consequences of prolonged or repeated admissions. Mental deterioration in the elderly is known to follow hospital admission in many instances and can therefore be minimized by a cautious admission policy, with use of alternatives whenever possible. Cognitive impairment in the elderly can also be reduced by avoidance of unnecessary medication and by the recognition of depression or infection.

2. Preventing chronic disability

Here the measures are aimed at reduction of chronic disability when disease or impairment have already occurred. These measures include:

(i) rehabilitation of patients with sensory and motor handicaps;

(ii) treatment of hypertension and of infections in the central nervous system, such as meningitis;

(iii) control of epilepsy and reduction of its secondary consequences, both physical and psychosocial;

(iv) combined treatment with medication and family care for

patients with schizophrenia (Jablensky *et al.* 1980; Falloon and Liberman 1983);

(v) the recognition and treatment of affective disorders. Here there is considerable scope for preventive action by making the diagnosis in the first place, as in patients with multiple somatic complaints who may be inappropriately investigated, or left untreated. Suicide is an obvious preventable consequence. The advent of lithium has contributed enormously to the lives of persons with recurrent affective disorder.

The World Health Organization report goes on to emphasize that, for full effectiveness, prevention programmes cannot stand on their own, but need to involve self-help groups, the media, cultural and religious forces, non-governmental organizations, and the provision of social support for families with afflicted members. Many governments do not have a national health policy in which there is a mental health component to provide a basis for these preventive activities.

It seems reasonable to conclude from the World Health Organization report that a sizeable body of knowledge does exist which awaits application; and that administrative action is now much needed to achieve this. The coming years are likely to see an expansion of intervention programmes in this field, accompanied where possible by evaluation of their impact.

8

The evaluation of services

What are the questions?; informative designs; need; criteria for measures of outcome; financial and non-financial costs; illustration using the evaluation of the Italian Law Reform; conclusion.

WHAT ARE THE QUESTIONS?

Services exist to reduce morbidity. Their evaluation must therefore be an assessment of how well they perform in this task. It is quite striking that evaluation of services is somehow a neglected area of research activity, despite the large sums of money and human effort invested in providing care for a nation's sick or disabled members. The area can be strongly advocated to the younger clinician or behavioural scientist for the rich scientific opportunities it offers, and for the practical value of one's research efforts, which are likely to lead to findings capable of being used directly by planners. Commonly-used variables in evaluation research are listed in Table 8.1.

A comprehensive overview of the area, describing its fundamental structure and basic principles, has been provided by Wing and Hailey (1972) and Wing and Häfner (1973). In these volumes, Wing points to the dependence of planners on having evaluative information if the design of a service is to have an informed basis. Wing (1972, 1973) summarizes the proper concerns of evaluation research in six questions:

1. How many people are in contact with the various services that already exist, what patterns of contact do they make, and what are the temporal trends in contact rates?
2. What are the needs of these individuals and of their relatives?
3. Are the services provided at present meeting these needs effectively and economically?
4. How many other people, not in touch with services, also have needs, and are these needs different from those of people already in contact?

Table 8.1 Commonly used variables in evaluation research

1. Volume of throughput (person, admissions, episodes, attendances)
2. Clinical or sociodemographic characteristics of the consumers
3. Modes of treatment or management employed
4. Duration of treatment
5. Outcome measures, including relapse rates, over specified periods of follow-up
6. New morbidity emerging during care
7. Mortality
8. Effects of the service on families, on the staff, and on other services
9. Utilization of personnel; levels of training; how staff actually spend their time
10. Measures of satisfaction in patients, relatives, and staff
11. Penetration: are many who deserve it not reaching the service?
12. Financial and non-financial costs

5. What new services, or modifications to existing services, are needed to cater for unmet needs?
6. When innovations in service are introduced, do they in fact help to reduce need?

Although these questions are disarmingly plain and succinct, each one calls for considerable effort to obtain the information required to answer it. The first can sometimes be tackled from data already available in a systematized form, as in regions where a case register exists. More often, it requires much tedious work to retrieve it. The evaluator and his consumers will probably want to know some important features of the present 'throughput'. Some of these, and the distinctions between them, include:

- –the number of persons, or episodes of illness, or admissions, or attendances in a defined period (e.g. studies of parasuicide based on the Edinburgh Register and described by Kreitman 1988);
- –the social and demographic features of consumers;
- –how patients reach the service, through what agency, and under what circumstances (e.g. Goldberg and Huxley 1980);

–the diagnostic groups to which patients are said to belong;
–what actually happens to patients in the course of their contact with services;
–what time is spent in direct contact with specified professional staff;
–the duration of treatment.

Still under the first of Wing's questions is the matter of what the service is intending to achieve. This is essentially the *containment of morbidity*, first in patients themselves, secondly in the patient's immediate family, and thirdly in the general community. Wing argues that there are three components in psychiatric morbidity, each relevant to the evaluation of a service: the biological or psychological abnormalities of the illness itself (such as symptoms); adverse attitudes or behaviour which are secondary to the disorder (such as social and work competence, or personal habits); and premorbid attributes which handicap the person now that he or she is ill (such as poor education or limited personality resources). These three components Wing sees as summing together to make what is called 'disability'. The appropriateness of the treatment or service being evaluated has clearly to be examined in relation to this profile of morbidity, and to the resulting overall disability arising from its three components.

DESIGNS WHICH ARE INFORMATIVE

The reader will readily appreciate that information on all of the parameters of a service listed above is essentially descriptive. That is, it describes the pattern of consumption, but it does not show whether this is useful. As Wing puts it, service descriptions show 'the cumulative results of clinical and administrative decisions without indicating whether they are the right ones'. A quantitative description, therefore, can be taken only as preparatory work for a more definitive investigation. Wherever possible, this should be undertaken by an independent group who has no axe to grind and hopefully not too many preconceptions.

It is at this stage, when an evaluative study moves past the stage of naturalistic description, that a large number of designs offer themselves. In practice, the choice amongst them will usually be determined by circumstances and resources. The volume edited by

Wing and Hailey (1972) provides a good introduction to the field, describing how studies were actually conducted in the evaluation of a psychiatric service. Wing (1972) sets out the range of designs which can be used. The options include the following:

1. *An epidemiological study* This could be of the same general population as the catchment area for the service, so that the morbidity detected may be compared with the morbidity which has reached that service. Alternatively, the epidemiological study could include all or most other services in the area relevant to mental health, so that a comparison may be made between those in the index service and those being treated in other settings, including general practice.

2. *Comparisons between services* This refers to the selection of a particular service to contrast with the index one. An example would be a comparison between hospital and community care for severe psychiatric disorders, where both services are already taking place with unrelated intake procedures and no random allocation of patients. An example is the comparison of two services in Sussex by Grad and Sainsbury (1968).

3. *Subgroup comparisons* Useful contrasts can be made *within* a service by comparing two or more groups, provided the data can be intelligently interpreted. The comparison by Wing and Brown (1961) of patients with schizophrenia in three mental hospitals is an example. A recurrent problem here, however, is that the groups may not have been matched to start with, as in severity of disorder at intake to the hospital or to the study.

4. *Natural experiments* These are valuable opportunities which emerge where, for some independent reason, a distinct change is introduced to the pattern of a service. An outstanding example is the introduction of mental health reform in Italy in 1978, whereby the admission of patients to mental hospitals was brought to an end (Tansella *et al.* 1987). We shall return to consider that later in the chapter. Under such serendipitous circumstances, it may be possible to compare the 'before and after' features of the service, making the assumption that the patients had comparable characteristics in the

first place. More rarely, it is possible to contrast the traditional with the new service at the same time, again assuming the two groups were truly comparable at intake.

5. *Controlled trials* These must be seen as the most desirable of all, because they conform to the rigorous experimental design of a drug trial, with the exception that they cannot be double-blind. Out of a single pool of patients, individuals are randomly allocated to two or more patterns of care. Appropriate assessment of symptoms and disability are made at intake and at later intervals. Measures of outcome can be elaborated as wished, to include measures such as satisfaction on the part of patient, relatives and staff, costs of the separate treatments, and long-term benefits of adverse sequelae. An example is the comparison of hospital and community treatment carried out by Hoult *et al.* (1981, 1984). Hoult and his colleagues randomly allocated 120 psychiatric patients to standard hospital care and after-care, or to comprehensive community treatment. Patients in the latter group were not admitted if it could be avoided. The project team provided them and their relatives with comprehensive, assertive and prolonged follow-up treatment backed by a 24-hour crisis service. Community treatment was associated with a clinically superior outcome and was considered more satisfactory both by the patients and their relatives. Such trials are not without serious practical difficulties, as in ensuring random allocation and unbiased assessment. Clarke and Cornish (1972) have given a useful review of these problems in *The controlled trial in institutional research.*

The desirability of replication must be stressed for evaluation studies, particularly in trials. This is most valuable of all when it is undertaken on a different geographical population by different investigators. If a particular type of service can thereby be shown to be superior to others, in two or more populations, this is persuasive for its superiority.

NEED

A distinction should be made between need, demand and utilization. Wing (1973, p. 7) uses the concise definitions of Matthew (1971):

> A need for medical care exists when an individual has an illness or disability for which there is effective and acceptable treatment or care. It can be defined either in terms of the type of illness or disability causing the need or of the

treatment or facilities for treatment required to meet it. A demand for care exists when an individual considers that he has a need and wishes to receive care. Utilization occurs when an individual actually receives care. Need is not necessarily expressed as demand and demand is not necessarily followed by utilization, while, on the other hand, there can be demand and utilization without real underlying need for the particular service used.

Wing notes that having established a need for care, it still has to be accorded a priority alongside other needs, an issue which is complex and has been largely ignored, yet it is a process which is open to systematic enquiry. The recent re-allocation of massive service and research funds for AIDS is a topical example.

In mental health care, the particular treatment or type of care given to a patient is in large part a matter of clinical judgement, together with the constraint of what is locally available (Bebbington, personal communication). In this way, patients with comparable needs can be placed in quite different treatments, both within and between geographical regions, though this process of allocation may be to some extent capricious.

Wing's third question: 'Are the services meeting the need effectively and economically?' calls for some clear thinking on how success is to be operationally defined. There may be different views on what success is, in the eyes of the administrators, the medical, nursing and other staff, the patients and families involved, and the community. It will usually be wise for the researchers to set up their own criteria, alongside the others. It is in examining what actually happens and what staff really do that evaluation research reaches its central, but most difficult task. Furthermore, it is at this stage that staff feel themselves under investigation. Here, Wing points out that views may be expressed which are different from the evaluator's. But the latter should be aware that he too is no longer disinterested, and will dislike having his views challenged just as much as the agency staff dislike being told they are not as successful in their work as they thought.

The fourth question in Wing's list concerns needs for services which are not being met. A central issue here is what professional service is most effective and least costly in meeting such need, where the latter is well-specified. With this information, it would be possible to deploy services most effectively to meet at least some of those unmet needs. Readers will find it useful to consider how such unmet need can be established in the first place. There are some uncertainties here. For example, it is quite clear that the morbidity found in community surveys, most of which is not in contact with services, cannot all be claimed as unmet need. It is known that many of the 'cases' identified in surveys are less severe and of much shorter duration than those who contact services. Most of them have not passed Goldberg's *1st filter* (Chapter 6), for reasons which are not at all clear. Yet there has been a tendency to use community prevalence estimates from surveys for this purpose; for example, Srole *et al.* (1962) did so in the Midtown Manhattan Study. A proportion of such morbidity is short-lived, even if it does reach 'case' level on cross-sectional interviews. It should be noted, though, that Surtees *et al.* (1986) found that about 40 per cent of the women they found to be Research Diagnostic Criteria (RDC) cases in their Edinburgh survey were still cases at follow-up one year later; and 47 per cent of these initial cases had sought help from their general practitioners in the previous six months. These findings bespeak a considerable need for mental health care, although not necessarily by psychiatrists.

Much useful work remains to be done on the outcome of psychiatric disorders presenting at the primary care level, whether unrecognized, treated by the general practitioner or others in that team, or referred to specialist services. A group who have come to deserve considerably more attention in primary care are the elderly. In his classic study, Williamson *et al.* (1964) showed that depression and dementia were poorly recognized by general practitioners among the elderly in their care. Macdonald (1986) has since studied the recognition of depression in the elderly in further detail, in a general practice setting, finding much better ascertainment. Nevertheless, need at this primary care level remains an important target for operational research to guide policy.

CRITERIA FOR MEASURES OF OUTCOME

1. *Symptom severity and duration* The severity of symptoms, or the length of time during which they persist, or are disabling, are commonly accepted criteria. But such outcomes are really arranged along a continuum, so that it is very important to have the criteria well specified and consistently applied. The point in time when assessment is made must also be decided. Short periods of some months, or even a year, may say rather little, because relapse may take place afterwards. The longer the time to which the outcome

measures refer, the more the study reveals about *therapeutic effects which are enduring*. The frequency of relapse should be built into the study wherever possible, so that outcome measures can reflect both success and failure.

2. *New morbidity and mortality* A truly comprehensive evaluation of services should include ascertainment of any fresh or additional morbidity, or excess mortality, which may be associated with the treatment. This is essentially the notion of *primum non nocere* (above all, do no harm) observed by good physicians since classical times. Secondary morbidity in the form of institutionalization was commonly found in mental hospitals. Such social and cognitive deterioration continues to occur in nursing homes and geriatric wards. Conceivably, morbidity in unexpected areas could *decrease*, so this too might be looked for. An example in pharmacology was the observation that iproniazid had an antidepressant as well as an antituberculous effect. More relevant in psychiatry, however, is vigilance to minimize the acquisition of social disabilities which are not primarily part of the disease. This was seen, for example, in the institutional neurosis described by Barton (1966), and in the social breakdown syndrome identified by Gruenberg (1974) (see Chapter 5, p. 107). It may be seen emerging today in the social environment which characterizes life in many nursing homes for the elderly, although this has not been well documented.

3. *Effects on families, staff, and other services* There are more than the patients to be considered when any treatment programme is in action. It may have some effect on relatives, one hopes, to diminish their burden. But relatives may also want to retain some responsibility, and may resent complete abrogation of this. Then again, the service being studied may have effects on the mental health of other family members, which differ from the effects on them of other services. The dependent variables may therefore have to be extended to include the health and well-being of persons other than the patients. This was done by Grad and Sainsbury (1968) in their comparison; and by Hoult *et al.* (1981, 1984) in their trial. This issue would also be relevant in evaluating services for elderly persons with dementia. It was deliberately included by Wells and Jorm (1987) in their pilot evaluation of a new dementia service introduced by the Uniting Church in Victoria, Australia. Allocation to this service or to

standard community care was randomized. They found that admission of elderly persons with dementia to in-patient care was followed by a striking decrease in the carers' level of psychological symptoms, and an increase in their well-being. These changes did not take place in those carers whose elderly relatives were given standard community care.

The staff are another group to consider in evaluating a service. Although it is not commonly included, the health and well-being of the personnel who provide the service is a very reasonable subject for investigation. This may include recruitment patterns, indices of motivation and involvement, and the frequency of absenteeism or resignations as evidence of 'burnout'. The latter is a syndrome of tiredness, irritability, and loss of interest in work, often accompanied by somatic symptoms. It is thought to be due to excessive psychological demands in the workplace, particularly in those exposed for long periods to people whose behaviour may be troubling, such as schoolchildren, psychiatric patients, the elderly, or prisoners. It seems to occur, or to be recognized, only in industrialized countries. An instrument for its measurement has been constructed and validated (Maslach and Jackson 1981; Iwanicki and Schwab 1981). The edited volume by Farber (1983) provides a commentary on the theoretical basis of burnout, its nature, treatment, and prevention.

One component in a service may influence the pattern of usage in other sectors. For example, attendance at a day hospital may reduce the frequency with which the patients call their family doctor. The principle to bear in mind here is that any particular service is only one part of a much larger system. To generate comprehensive and practically useful information, an evaluative study may have to include some of these wider issues.

Wing's fifth and sixth questions deal with changes or innovations to services. He sees these as part of a continuing cycle of new planning and new evaluation, whereby the ultimate aim is the development of services that are responsible (for health care of a population), comprehensive (in the range of services available), and integrated (in the communication taking place between the elements of the service).

FINANCIAL AND NON-FINANCIAL COSTS

The costs of a service are often the single variable which dominates the thinking of administrators and policy makers. To make a comprehensive estimate of such costs is a complicated task, sometimes requiring collaboration with a health economist. However, by thinking through the various components which incur expenditure, a clinician can arrive at a realistic estimate. An example is the study by Andrews *et al.* (1985) on the costs of schizophrenia (see also Chapter 5, p. 121). The cost of providing a service is one issue; but there will often be other important costs, as in lost earnings by the patient and his relatives, and in pensions received.

By non-financial costs is meant those consequences to the patient and his family which cannot be expressed in monetary terms, but which may have a sizeable impact on their quality of life. An outstanding example is the work of Annalise Dupont (1986) on the effect on families of caring for a severely retarded child (see Chapter 5, p. 119), or of Grad and Sainsbury (1968) on the effect on relatives of community care. A literature is beginning to develop on the evaluation of psychiatric services with a cost–benefit component. This is becoming a growth area in psychiatric research, and should be recognized as one which offers a number of attractions, including some challenges in methodology. The papers by Glass and Goldberg (1977) and Goldberg and Jones (1980) provide a good starting point, because they clarify what is meant by analyses of cost–benefit and cost-effectiveness. Glass and Goldberg conclude that: 'The advantage of cost–benefit study . . . is that it allows an explicit judgement to be made about whether the extra quality (of one service) is worth the extra price by providing consistent information about the difference in quality and price . . . '. They also point out something which is particularly appealing: 'the process of formulating an analysis of this kind can lead to the generation of alternatives to the original services which one sets out to compare alternatives which may combine the virtues of the two services but achieve a higher ratio of effectiveness to cost'.

THE EVALUATION OF PSYCHIATRIC REFORM IN ITALY

We now consider a natural experiment in psychiatric services which may come to be seen as one of the more remarkable events in the history of caring for the mentally ill. It is worthwhile examining because of its unusual nature and administrative significance. In May 1978, the Italian Parliament passed Law 180, which brought to an end the use of mental hospitals in the care of persons with psychiatric disorders. World-wide interest in the so-called Italian Reform has arisen because of at least three factors: its political origins, arising largely from the left; curiosity outside Italy to see its consequences; and the scientific opportunities it has afforded as a true natural experiment in mental health care. The events and the outcome to date have been reviewed by Tansella and Williams (1987). Further information derived from the case register in Verona has been provided by Zimmermann-Tansella *et al.* (1985) and Burti *et al.* (1986).

The essence of the Italian Reform was that strong criticism of conditions in mental hospitals had arisen, endorsed by left-wing political parties. Such criticism was almost certainly justified by the conditions then prevailing in mental hospitals. A national referendum became imminent, and could have led to enforced resignation of the Italian Government. To prevent this, the Parliament passed Law 180. This had five main provisions: first admissions to mental hospitals were stopped after May 1978, and *any* admission after December 1981; 15-bed psychiatric units in general hospitals were to be set up; community psychiatric services for defined catchment areas were to be established; compulsory admission to the general hospital units could be authorized by a mayor or his designate, on the basis of two medical recommendations; and both the general hospital units and the community services were to be staffed by existing personnel.

In determining what the consequences have been, the two main questions are the extent to which these changes have actually been implemented, and how well they work (Tansella and Williams 1987). As might be anticipated, the answer to both questions varies across regions, the gradient being mainly from north to south. In the latter, the law has probably not been fully implemented, though there is a gradual shift from mental hospital to community care. For true evaluation, based on data about the operation of services rather than impression, the best evidence comes from areas where community services have been developing for sometime, and particularly where case registers have been running since *before* the new law. First, three case registers, in Lomest, South Verona, and Portogruaro, show that there has been a high level of success in moving towards community-oriented services, although this was already starting before the reform. Secondly, there is no evidence that *new* long-stay in-patients have accumulated. Thirdly, compulsory admission has decreased substantially; there were actually none in Portogruaro in 1984. Some observers thought that the utilization of private psychiatric beds would increase, but Tansella *et al.* (1986) found no evidence for this when they examined reliable national data. Private beds have actually decreased in number.

Williams *et al.* (1986*b*) examined trends in suicide rates across all regions of Italy before and since the reform. They found that rates had increased, mainly in the north central regions. The increase correlated negatively with the provision of psychiatric beds in general hospitals. The latter is likely to be an indicator of the availability of more general psychiatric resources. The reduction in mental hospital beds following the Italian reform was unrelated to changes in the suicide rate.

Tansella and Williams conclude that where the reform has been implemented, the Italian model of community care, without use of mental hospitals, is able to care for all the psychiatric disorders that arise in a community. These authors emphasize the central role which general practitioners can play in providing primary medical care to mentally disabled people. Once again we see that the general practitioner is well placed to ensure that the other, non-medical resources of the health care team are effectively deployed. Clearly, a great deal has been learned from these studies about the operation of psychiatric services in meeting needs, particularly for those with severe mental disorders. It is still too early, however, to know the long-term consequences of the reform, for individuals, and for the Italian community and its services.

CONCLUSION

The components of evaluation set out here, based on the introduction to the field by Wing (1973), provides a basic structure. These will allow the reader to pursue his interests, perhaps tackling a particular theme where an opportunity has emerged, without losing sight of the whole. It is helpful to recall the statement at the beginning of the chapter, that services exist to reduce morbidity; and that must remain the ultimate yardstick for their evaluation.

9
Synthesis

Measurement of morbidity; measurement of social factors; properties of the individual.

We can now ask what general statements social psychiatry is able to make about mental disorders, and where further research efforts are likely to be best directed. From the body of knowledge now assembled, one can see that a single paradigm has dominated thinking: that an examination of the social environment, and of particular types of experience in life, will provide an explanation for many mental disorders. Such a paradigm carries the expectation that social factors can be shown to play a major role in both the onset and course of mental disorders. This expectation has not been fulfilled. The contribution of the social environment to aetiology, whether for the psychoses or for minor psychiatric disorders, has not been as powerful as expected. There are indeed events and experiences which are aetiologically significant. Some of these exert effects after very long intervals, others within only hours. But the effects are not invariable; some individuals succumb, yet often a majority appear unscathed. In short, some persons are more vulnerable to adversity than others.

This vulnerability can be contextual, whereby there is some interaction between a particular experience and other situational factors, external to the person; or it can be intrapersonal, whereby some individuals are intrinsically more likely than others to respond to some environments by developing psychological symptoms or a psychiatric disorder. Such intrapersonal vulnerability may be explicitly biological, as in genetic predisposition; or it may lie in personality traits which render the person susceptible to, say, depression (Foulds 1965). Finally, it is incontrovertible that psychological attributes of the individual have much to do with the impact of environmental experiences; and this *interaction* between the two sets of risk factors may be more powerful than either the environmental experience or the personal attributes themselves. We have also seen in Chapter 4 that properties of the individual, including both personality and sociodemographic factors, may determine to a considerable extent what environmental exposures the person is likely to have in the first place. People are to a large extent the architects of their social environment.

What is unarguable is the powerful influence of the social environment *on the course* of mental disorders and on what actually happens to individuals after they have become ill. This takes our consideration directly to the use of social psychiatric knowledge for treatment, and for secondary or tertiary prevention. Clearly, this is an underdeveloped area which now calls for much more attention, because these are the delivery points for all knowledge we have gained about the aetiology and course of disorders.

In the last three decades, the priorities facing the aetiological side of social psychiatry have been to develop valid and reliable measures of psychiatric disorders, with valid and reliable measures of social variables to be related to them. There should now be added a third: the need for some new hypotheses on aetiology. Social psychiatry has had a fair mileage out of sociodemographic variables, the life-event hypothesis, and other experiential factors. A new paradigm is now much needed. A change to be advocated is in the number of domains typically considered in aetiological research. Throughout its history, social psychiatry has usually chosen to work with only two sets of variable: morbidity and social factors. This has been the case in most research on sociodemographic variables, where it is a reasonable starting point for exploration; but it can also be seen in the life-event industry, where personality or some attention to contextual factors have been late in having their importance recognized. This oversight, with its implicit neglect of aetiological factors in the intrapsychic and neurobiological domains, may have been due to too great a separation between social psychiatry and clinical practice. Clinicians know better than to attend exclusively to social factors when trying to understand the genesis of a patient's illness. But social psychiatry seems repeatedly to have assessed only environmental factors in individuals' current or earlier lives with the expectation of finding substantial causal effects. It should not be surprising that only weak associations have been found. Where effects do appear to be present, there is usually a high likelihood that the social variable is confounded by factors in another domain, particularly in the broad category of intrapersonal properties. These should be seen as including both personality traits and biological attributes. There are therefore three domains to consider in psychiatric epidemiology: the disorder, the past and present social environment, and properties of the individual. We shall consider each of these in turn.

THE MEASUREMENT OF MORBIDITY

For the measurement of morbidity, we have seen the considerable advances made through the introduction of standardized diagnostic criteria, accompanied by standardized case-finding instruments. Criteria which are both capable of being widely used and likely to be valid are the cornerstone of any research which requires homogeneity in its case material. But problems remain. For example, the diagnosis of depression is still untidy, in that different classificatory systems do not relate easily to each other, and identify different individuals as cases. There is so far no satisfactory way to accommodate states of mixed depression and anxiety, although these are commonly encountered in primary care. Until a non-invasive biological test is available, the diagnosis of dementia presents some formidable problems for international studies, particularly in the important matters of diagnosing mild dementia and accurately identifying cases of Alzheimer's disease in elderly populations. These remaining tasks illustrate that, although measurement of morbidity has progressed very greatly, there is much scope for further contributions.

The validation of nosological classes, whether these be in the ICD or DSM systems, has proved to be very difficult (Jablensky 1985; Henderson 1985). There is usually no satisfactory gold standard. Meanwhile, we can anticipate useful progress with the new revisions of these systems. Attention will now be focused on the forthcoming ICD–10 Clinical Guidelines and its Diagnostic Criteria for Research; and on DSM-III-R from the United States. Both have much in common in their structure and content. The ICD–10 for Mental Disorders represents a considerable achievement in fundamental thinking balanced by international consultations. Clearly, not everyone will be comfortable in using it, but as a step forward in scientific psychiatry which is also closely related to the delivery of better services, ICD–10 provides an attractive agenda for research.

Obtaining reliable and valid case-histories

Interview instruments such as the Present State Examination (PSE), and now the Schedule for Clinical Assessment in Neuropsychiatry

(SCAN), Diagnostic Interview Schedule (DIS), Composite International Diagnostic Interview (CIDI), or Schedule for Affective Disorders and Schizophrenia (Lifetime version) (SADS–L), are designed to obtain information on recent symptoms and behaviour, and to allow the respondent to be allocated to a diagnostic category within the ICD or DSM systems. In the last three of these instruments, information on previous experience of such phenomena is also sought. Indeed, as we have seen, this 'history' can be extended to a lifetime, by asking the quetion, 'Have you ever . . . ?', then making the hazardous attempt to date the onset and duration of the episode.

In clinical practice, however, there are at least three further components in obtaining a comprehensive case history. First, the history of onset is frequently of great value in making a diagnosis. For example, it is mandatory in assessing the significance of cognitive impairment in an elderly person. An attempt to obtain a history of onset in a standardized manner has been made in an adjunct to recently developed instruments. It is an integral part of the History and Aetiology Schedule of the Geriatric Mental State Examination by Copeland and his colleagues (Copeland *et al.* 1976, 1986*a*, *b* 1988); and of the CAMDEX interview for the elderly (Roth *et al.* 1986). The yield in explanatory power is likely to be considerable if such systems are now used in epidemiological field surveys, where aetiology is a major objective.

The second component is a history of previous episodes. Although a clinician would invariably enquire about these in trying to determine the causes of a patient's illness and its prognosis, epidemiological field surveys have typically focused only on current mental state, or changes in this during the period of a prospective study. Where attempts have been made to determine past history, some problems in validity have emerged (Gershon and Guroff 1984), but these do not seem insuperable. Aetiology cannot be tackled using only cross-sectional data, but self-reports of life-time prevalence, as obtained in the Epidemiologic Catchment Area (ECA) studies, call for cautious interpretation.

A third component is information on the person's premorbid personality in terms of prominent traits, in contrast to evidence of personality disorder. This is technically very demanding and it is quite separate from the primary objectives of intruments such as the PSE or DIS. Yet it is a well-established part of a comprehensive clinical case history, and it is recognized by clinicians as important for aetiology and management. Epidemiologists, however, have rarely been able to include this in their studies. An exception exists in the evaluation of personality according to the Sjöbring classification in the Lundby study by Hagnell and his colleagues (e.g. Hagnell 1966; Hagnell *et al.* 1973).

Measurement of social factors

The need here is to consolidate what has already been achieved. As we have seen, social factors are of three types: sociodemographic variables, which are a useful starting point, but can only be coarse representations of actual social experiences; early and late experiential factors. These can be postulated to be either beneficial, such as good parenting in childhood or plentiful social support in the present; or adverse, such as parental deprivation or recent adverse life-events. It is difficult to see how a new paradigm about social experience could be constructed in addition to these, as they seem jointly exhaustive.

Most of the measurement tools developed, such as for life-events, social support, or early experiences, are based on self-report. This is a grave deficiency. In Chapter 4, we examined the evidence about parental style generated by the Parental Bonding Instrument and the EMBU, where attempts have been made to overcome the effects of biased self-reports. This exemplifies the central importance of working with valid information if knowledge about aetiology is to be advanced in the domain of personal experiences. For life-events, the Bedford College method has no equal, but it is technically demanding. This means, quite simply, that adversity cannot be measured without the investment of considerable resources and training. No short-cut is methodologically satisfactory. The measurement of social support is in no better state. There, the priorities are to clarify what facets of the concept are likely to be relevant; then to choose and construct an instrument to measure them, preferably not only by self-report; to have measures of what support was actually received at the time of personal crisis, as advocated by Brown and his colleagues (Brown *et al.* 1986*a*); and finally, to be able to measure support unconfounded by personality.

Distinguishing between personal and social variables

The relationship between social or experiential factors on the one hand, and the onset or course of mental disorders on the other, has now been thoroughly studied. This large and important body of research can confidently claim to have shown that people do influence the mental health of others; and that many psychiatric disorders have an increased likelihood of occurring, or relapsing, when personal relationships are impaired. It has, however, proved consistently difficult to separate social or experiential factors from the personality characteristics of both the individual and those who make up his or her social environment. Social factors are, after all, reducible to actual behaviours, either in the present or in the person's developmental years. These behaviours are dictated at least in part by the recipient's personality and temperament. We noted in Chapter 4 that persons with high neuroticism scores have an increased probability of experiencing adverse life-events. Experiential factors are thereby influenced by personality. We have held that the same may hold for the level of social support available to a person, particularly from close personal relationships.

The implications for further research are far reaching. An enquiry that sets out to investigate a social factor ought ideally to include simultaneous assessment of personality and temperament. To omit this is to omit a major component in the aetiological equation. The implications for intervention or preventive action are equally compelling: rather than attempt to change a person's immediate social environment directly, it may be wiser to strive after changes in that person's social behaviour. The challenge now facing the discipline is to have a much better understanding of this interface between the person and his social environment. There is an opportunity here for some innovative thinking, to develop a theory-driven basis for such exploration. For example, there is promise in recent work on the fit or congruence between a person's habitual cognitive style and his or her current social environment (Power and Champion 1986; Power 1987).

PROPERTIES OF THE INDIVIDUAL

After constructing measures of morbidity and of the social environment, psychiatric epidemiology needs to tackle what can be denoted collectively as the third domain: properties of the individual. These may be in the large area of personality; or in other psychological attributes, such as cognitive style and habitual defence or coping mechanisms. Some of the traits which may increase vulnerability to non-psychotic psychiatric disorders are: neuroticism, low self-esteem, locus of control, interpersonal dependency, low ego-strength, egocentricity, and intropunitiveness. But there is another group, also a property of the individual; these are biological characteristics, and are to be found in measures of brain function and of both brain and general metabolism.

If it is acknowledged that social factors produce only weak causal effects, and that there is quite remarkable variation between individuals, then certain properties of these individuals now need to be identified, which may account for these differences. If these properties are not mainly in a person's social and interpersonal circumstances, they must be psychological or biological. This presents a formidable challenge, because measures of personality and of biological attributes are for the most part unsuited for use in epidemiological field surveys. But these technical hindrances should not be seen from the outset as insurmountable. The over-riding objective is to expand the horizon of psychiatric epidemiology beyond the social environment. It now has to understand much more about host resistance.

This latter term is itself now outdated, because resistance or susceptibility, as we have seen in these pages, are rarely determined by nature or nurture acting alone but are a product of the interaction of these. For this reason, the very term social psychiatry may be deficient because it does not accurately reflect how we should think about mental disorders and go about our business. Sartorius (1988) has gone so far as to predict that 'social psychiatry will disappear and it is likely that this world will be a slightly better place without it'. He argues that the concerns of social psychiatry will not lose their importance, but will come to be handled in the broader context of clinical practice. By holding to an expanded, interactionist paradigm, psychiatric epidemiology can continue to accord close attention to social factors, *inter alia*. It will thereby augment its already considerable contribution to the relief of mental disorders, and the promotion of public health.

References

Ackerman, N.W. (1966). *Treating the troubled family*. Basic Books, New York.

Åkesson, H.O. (1969). A population study of senile and arteriosclerotic psychoses. *Human Heredity*, **19**, 546–66.

Alloway, R., and Bebbington P. (1987). The buffer theory of social support—a review of the literature. *Psychological Medicine*, **17**, 91–108.

Amaducci, L.A., Rocca W.A., and Schoenberg, B.S. (1986). Origin of the distinction between Alzheimer's disease and senile dementia: how history can clarify nosology. *Neurology*, **36**, 1497–9.

American Psychiatric Association (1980). *Diagnostic and statistical manual of mental disorders*, 3rd edn, DSM-III. Division of Public Affairs, American Psychiatric Association, Washington.

Andrews, G., and Tennant, C. (1978*a*). Life events, stress and psychiatric illness: a review. *Psychological Medicine*, **8**, 545–9.

Andrews, G., and Tennant, C. (1978*b*). Being upset and becoming ill: an appraisal of the relation between life events and physical illness. *Medical Journal of Australia*, **1**, 324–7.

Andrews, G., Hall, W., Goldstein, G., Lapsley, H., Bartels, R., and Silove, D. (1985). The economic costs of schizophrenia. *Archives of General Psychiatry*, **42**, 537–43.

Anthony, J.C. (1988). Case-control studies. In *Handbook of social psychiatry* (ed. A.S. Henderson and G.D. Burrows). Elsevier, Amsterdam.

Antonovsky, A., Maoz, B., Dowty N., and Wijsenbeek, H. (1971). Twenty-five years later: a limited study of the sequelae of the concentration camp experience. *Social Psychiatry*, **6**, 186–93.

Arey, S., and Warheit, G.J. (1980). Psychosocial costs of living with psychologically disturbed family members. In *The social consequences of psychiatric illness* (ed. L.N. Robins, P.J. Clayton, and J.K. Wing), pp. 158–75. Brunner Mazel, New York.

Armitage, P., and Berry G. (1987). *Statistical methods in medical research*, 2nd edn. Blackwell Scientific Publications, Oxford.

Arrindell W.A. *et al.* (1986*a*). Cross-national generalizability of patterns of parental rearing behavior: invariance of EMBU dimensional representations of healthy subjects from Australia, Denmark, Hungary, Italy, and The Netherlands. *Personality and Individual Differences*, **7**, 103–12.

Arrindell, W.A., Perris, C., Perris, M., Eisemann, M., Van Der Ende, J., and Von Knorring, L. (1986*b*). Cross-national invariance of dimensions of parental rearing behaviour: comparison of psychometric data of Swedish depressives and healthy subjects with Dutch target ratings on the EMBU. *British Journal of Psychiatry*, **148**, 305–9.

Aschaffenburg, G. (Ed.) (1915). *Handbuch der Psychiatrie*. Deuticke, Leipzig.

Bacon, F. (1965). Essay 27—Of friendship. In *Francis Bacon. A selection of his works* (ed. S. Warhaft), pp. 112–19. Macmillan, Toronto.

Bagley, C. (1968). The evaluation of a suicide prevention scheme by an ecological method. *Social Science and Medicine*, **2**, 1–14.

Bagley, C. (1973). Occupational class and symptoms of depression. *Social Science and Medicine*, **7**, 327–40.

Banks, M.M., and Jackson, P.R. (1982). Unemployment and risk of minor psychiatric disorder in young people: cross-sectional and longitudinal evidence. *Psychological Medicine*, **12**, 789–98.

Barnes, J.A. (1954). Class and committees in a Norwegian island parish. *Human Relations*, **7**, 39–58.

Barraclough, B.M. (1969). The effect that coroners have on the suicide rate and the open verdict rate. In *Psychiatric epidemiology* (ed. E.H. Hare and J.K. Wing), pp. 361–5. Oxford University Press.

Barraclough B.M. (1973). Differences between national suicide rates. *British Journal of Psychiatry*, **122**, 95–6.

Barraclough, B., and Hughes, J. (1987). *Suicide. Clinical and epidemiological studies*. Croom Helm, London.

Bartlett, F.C. (1932). *Remembering: A study of experimental and social psychology*. Cambridge University Press.

Barton, R. (1966). *Institutional neurosis*. Wright, Bristol.

Bartrop, R.W., and Porritt, D. (1988). Biological sequelae of adverse experiences. In *Handbook of social psychiatry* (ed. A.S. Henderson and G.D. Burrows). Elsevier, Amsterdam.

Bebbington, P. (1980). Causal models and logical inference in epidemiological psychiatry. *British Journal of Psychiatry*, **136**, 317–25.

Bebbington, P. (1985). Psychosocial aetiology of schizophrenia and affective disorders. In *Psychiatry* (ed. R. Michels). Lippincot, Philadelphia.

Bebbington, P.E. (1987*a*). Marital status and depression: a study of English national admission statistics. *Acta Psychiatrica Scandinavica*, **75**, 640–50.

Bebbington, P.E. (1987*b*). Life events in schizophrenia. The World Health Organization Collaborative Study. *Social Psychiatry*, **22**, 179–80.

Bebbington, P.E. (1988). The social epidemiology of clinical depression. In *Handbook of studies in social psychiatry* (ed. A.S. Henderson and G.D. Burrows). Elsevier, Amsterdam.

Bebbington, P., Hurry, J., Tennant, C., Sturt, E., and Wing, J.K. (1981*a*). Epidemiology of mental disorders in Camberwell. *Psychological Medicine*, **11**, 1–19.

Bebbington, P.E., Tennant, C., and Hurry, J. (1981*b*). Adversity and the nature of psychiatric disorder in the community. *Journal of Affective Disorders*, **3,** 345–66.

Bebbington, P., Tennant, C., Sturt, E., and Hurry, J. (1984). The domain of life events: a comparison of two techniques of description. *Psychological Medicine*, **14,** 219–22.

Bebbington P.E. *et al.* (1988). The Camberwell Collaborative Depression Study. I. Depressed probands: adversity and the form of depression. *British Journal of Psychiatry*, in press.

Beck, A.T. (1967). *Depression: Clinical, experimental, and theoretical aspects*. Harper and Row, New York.

Beck, A.T. (1976). *Cognitive therapy and the emotional disorders*. Meridian, New York.

Beck, A.T., Rush, A.J., Shaw, B.F., and Emergy, G. (1979). *Cognitive therapy of depression: A treatment manual*. Guilford, New York.

Bedford, A., and Foulds, G.A. (1978). *Manual of the Delusions-Symptoms States Inventory* (*State of Anxiety-Depression*). NFER, Windsor.

Bennett, D.H. (1978). Social forms of psychiatric treatment. In *Schizophrenia: Towards a new synthesis* (ed. J.K. Wing), pp. 211–31. Academic Press, London.

Bentovim, A. (1986). Family therapy when the child is the referred patient. In *An introduction to the psychotherapies*, 2nd edn (ed. S. Bloch), pp. 198–221. Oxford University Press.

Berg, I., Consterdine, M., Hullin, R., McGuire, R., and Tyrer, S. (1978). The effect of two randomly allocated court procedures on truancy. *British Journal of Criminology*, **18,** 232–44.

Bergmann, K., Kay, D.W.K., Foster, E.M., McKechnie, A.A., and Roth, M. (1971). A follow-up study of randomly selected community residents to assess the effects of chronic brain syndrome and cerebrovascular disease. In *New prospects in the study of mental disorders in old age*, pp. 856–65. Excerpta Medica, Amsterdam.

Berkman, L.F. (1986). Social networks, support, and health: taking the next step forward. *American Journal of Epidemiology*, **123,** 559–62.

Berkman, L.F., and Syme, S.L. (1979). Social networks, host resistance and mortality. A nine year follow up study of Alameda County residents. *American Journal of Epidemiology*, **109,** 186–204.

Berkson, J. (1946). Limitations of the application of fourfold table analysis to hospital data. *Biometrics Bulletin*, **2,** 47–53.

Birley, J.L.T., and Brown, G.W. (1968). Crises and life changes preceding the onset or relapse of acute schizophrenia: clinical aspects. *British Journal of Psychiatry*, **116,** 327–33.

Birtchnell, J. (1970). Early parent death and mental illness. *British Journal of Psychiatry*, **116,** 281–8.

Birtchnell, J. (1971). Social class, parental social class, and social mobility in psychiatric patients and general population controls. *Psychological Medicine*, **1,** 209–21.

Birtchnell, J. (1980). Women whose mothers died in childhood: an outcome study. *Psychological Medicine*, **10,** 699–713.

Birtchnell, J. (1984). Dependence and its relationship to depression. *British Journal of Medical Psychology*, **57,** 215–25.

Blazer, D.G. (1983). Impact of late-life depression on the social network. *American Journal of Psychiatry*, **140,** 162–6.

Blazer D. *et al.* (1985). Psychiatric disorders: a rural/urban comparison. *Archives of General Psychiatry*, **42,** 651–6.

Bloch, S., and Crouch, E. (1985). *Therapeutic factors in group psychotherapy.* Oxford University Press.

Blomfield, J.M., and Douglas, J.W.B. (1956). Bedwetting—prevalence among children aged 4–7 years. *Lancet*, **1,** 850–2.

Bloom, B.L., Hodges, W.F., Kern, M.B., and McFadden, S.C. (1985). A preventive intervention programme for the newly separated. *American Journal of Orthopsychiatry*, **55,** 9–26.

Bollerup, T.R. (1975). Prevalence of mental illness among 70-year-olds domiciled in nine Copenhagen suburbs. *Acta Psychiatrica Scandinavica*, **51,** 327–39.

Böök, J.A. (1953). A genetic and neuropsychiatric investigation of a North Swedish population. *Acta Genetica*, **4,** 345–414.

Böök, J.A., Wetterbergh, L., Modrzewska, K. and Unge, C. (1978). Schizophrenia in a North Swedish population, 1900–75. *Clinical Genetics*, **13,** 110.

Bowlby, J. (1969). *Attachment and loss*, Vol. 1: *Attachment*. Hogarth Press, London.

Bowlby J. (1973). *Attachment and loss*, Vol. 2: *Separation: Anxiety and anger*. Hogarth Press, London.

Bowlby, J. (1977*a*). The making and breaking of affectional bonds. I. Aetiology and psychopathology in the light of attachment theory. *British Journal of Psychiatry*, **130,** 201–10.

Bowlby, J. (1977*b*). The making and breaking of affectional bonds. II. Some principles of psychotherapy. *British Journal of Psychiatry*, **130,** 421–31.

Bowlby, J. (1980). *Attachment and loss*, Vol. 3: *Loss, sadness and depression*. Hogarth Press, London.

Boyd, J.H., and Weissman, M. (1981). Epidemiology of affective disorders. *Archives of General Psychiatry*, **38,** 1039–46.

Boyden, S. (1969). The impact of civilization on human biology. *Australian Journal of Experimental Biology and Medical Science*, **47,** 287–98.

Boyden, S. (1972). The environment and human health. *Medical Journal of Australia*, **1,** 1229–34.

Boyden, S. (1980). The need for an holistic approach to human health and well-being. In *Changing disease patterns and human behaviour* (ed. N.F. Stanley and R.A. Joske), pp. 622–44. Academic Press, Sydney.

Boyden, S. (1987). *Western civilization in biological perspective.* Oxford Science Publications.

Braithwaite, V.A. (1987). Coming to terms with burden in home care. *Australian Journal of Ageing*, **6,** 20–3.

Brewer, C., and Lait, J. (1980). *Can social work survive*? Temple Smith, London.

Brewin, C. (1980). Explaining the lower rates of psychiatric treatment among Asian immigrants to the United Kingdom: a preliminary study. *Social Psychiatry*, **15,** 17–19.

Bridges, K.W., and Goldberg, D.P. (1985). Somatic presentation of DSM-III psychiatric disorders in primary care. *Journal of Psychosomatic Research*, **29,** 563–9.

Briscoe, M. (1982). Sex differences in psychological well-being. *Psychological Medicine, Monograph Supplement 1*, 1–46.

Broadhead, W.E. *et al.* (1983). The epidemiologic evidence for a relationship between social support and health. *American Journal of Epidemiology*, **117,** 521–37.

Broadhurst, A. (1972). Clinical psychology and the general practitioner. *British Medical Journal*, **1,** 793–5.

Brodaty, H., and Andrews, G. (1983). Brief psychotherapy in family practice. A controlled prospective intervention trial. *British Journal of Psychiatry*, **143,** 11–19.

Broe, G.A., Akhtar, A.J., Andrews, G.R., Caird, F.I., Gilmore, A.J.J., and McLennan, W.J. (1976). Neurological disorders in the elderly at home. *Journal of Neurology, Neurosurgery and Psychiatry*, **39,** 362–66.

Brown, G.W. (1981). Life events, psychiatric disorder and physical illness. *Journal of Psychosomatic Research*, **25,** 461–73.

Brown, G.W., and Birley, J.L.T. (1968). Crises and life changes and the onset of schizophrenia. *Journal of Health and Social Behaviour*, **9,** 203–14.

Brown, G.W., and Harris, T. (1978). *Social origins of depression: A study of psychiatric disorder in women.* Tavistock, London.

Brown, G.W., and Harris, T. (1986). Stressor, vulnerability and depression: a question of replication. *Psychological Medicine*, **16,** 739–44.

Brown, G.W., and Rutter, M.L. (1966). The measurement of family activities and relationships. *Human Relations*, **19,** 241–63.

Brown, G.W., Carstairs, G.M., and Topping, G.C. (1958). The post hospital adjustment of chronic mental patients. *Lancet*, **2,** 685–9.

Brown, G.W., Monck, E.M., Carstairs, G.M., and Wing, J.K. (1962). Influence of family life on the course of schizophrenic illness. *British Journal of Preventive and Social Medicine*, **16,** 55–68.

Brown, G.W., Bone, M., Dalison, B., and Wing, J.K. (1966). *Schizophrenia and social care*. Oxford University Press.

Brown, G.W., Birley, J.L.T., and Wing, J.K. (1972). Influence of family life on the course of schizophrenic disorders: a replication. *British Journal of Psychiatry*, **121,** 241–58.

Brown, G.W., Sklair, F., Harris, T.O., and Birley, J.L.T. (1973). Life events and psychiatric disorders. I. Some methodological issues. *Psychological Medicine*, **3,** 74–87.

Brown, G.W., Bhrolcháin, M.N., and Harris, T. (1975). Social class and psychiatric disturbance among women in an urban population. *Sociology*, **9,** 225–54.

Brown, G.W., Davidson, S., Harris, T., Maclean, U., Pollock, S., and Prudo, R. (1977). Psychiatric disorder in London and North Uist. *Social Science and Medicine*, **11,** 367–77.

Brown, G.W., Andrews, B., Harris, T., Adler, Z., and Bridge, L. (1986*a*). Social support, self-esteem and depression. *Psychological Medicine*, **16,** 813–31.

Brown, G.W., Bifulco, A., Harris, T., and Bridge, L. (1986*b*). Life stress, chronic subclinical symptoms and vulnerability to clinical depression. *Journal of Affective Disorders*, **11,** 1–19.

Brugha, T. *et al.* (1982). Social networks, attachments and support in minor affective disorders: a replication. *British Journal of Psychiatry*, **141,** 249–55.

Bruun, K. *et al.* (1975). *Alcohol control policies in public health perspective*. Finnish Foundation for Alcohol Studies, Helsinki.

Buglass, D., Dugard, P., and Kreitman, N. (1970). Multiple standardization of parasuicide ('attempted suicide') rates in Edinburgh. *British Journal of Preventive and Social Medicine*, **24,** 182–6.

Burti, L., Garzotto, N., Siciliani, O., Zimmermann-Tansella, C., and Tansella, M. (1986). South Verona's psychiatric service: an integrated system of community care. *Hospital and Community Psychiatry*,. **37,** 809–13.

Carstairs, G.M., and Kapur, R.L. (1976). *The great universe of Kota: Stress, change and mental disorder in an Indian village*. Hogarth Press, London.

Cassel, J. (1976). The contribution of the social environment to host resistance. *American Journal of Epidemiology*, **104,** 107–23.

Chick, J. (1982). Epidemiology of alcohol use and its hazards. *Medical Bulletin*, **38,** 3–8.

Chowdhury, N., and Kreitman, N. (1971). A comparison of parasuicides ('attempted suicide') and the clients of the telephone Samaritan service. *Applied Social Studies*, **3,** 51–7.

Clare, A.W., and Corney, R.H. (eds) (1982). *Social work and primary health care*. Academic Press, London.

Clark, D.F. (1979). The clinical psychologist in primary care. *Social Science and Medicine,* **13A,** 707–13.

Clarke, R.V.G., and Cornish, D.B. (1972). *The controlled trial in institutional research—Paradigm or pitfall for penal evaluers.* Home Office Research Studies, No. 15. HMSO, London.

Clausen, J.A., and Yarrow, M.R. (1955). Paths to the mental hospital. *Journal of Social Issues*, **2,** 25–32.

Clayton, P.J. (1974). Mortality and morbidity in the first year of widowhood. *Archives of General Psychiatry*, **30,** 747–50.

Clayton, P.J. (1979). The sequelae and nonsequelae of conjugal bereavement. *American Journal of Psychiatry*, **136,** 1530–34.

Clayton, P.J. (1981). The epidemiology of bipolar affective disorder. *Comprehensive Psychiatry*, **22,** 31–43.

Clayton, P.J. (1982). Bereavement. In *Handbook of affective disorders* (ed. E.S. Paykel), pp. 403–15. Churchill Livingstone, London.

Cohen, J. (1968). Weighted kappa: nominal scale agreement with provision for scaled disagreement of partial credit. *Psychological Bulletin*, **70,** 213–20.

Cohn, R.M. (1978). The effect of employment status change on self attitudes. *Social Psychology*, **41,** 81–93.

Cooley, C.H. (1909). *Social organization: A study of the larger mind.* C. Scribner's Sons, New York.

Cooper, B. (1981). Psychiatric illness in general medical practice. An investigation in Mannheim. *International Journal of Rehabilitation Research*, **4,** 86–7.

Cooper, B. (1984). Home and away: the disposition of mentally ill old people in an urban population. *Social Psychiatry*, **19,** 187–96.

Cooper, B., and Bickel, H. (1984). Population screening and the early detection of dementing disorders in old age: a review. *Psychological Medicine*, **14,** 81–95.

Cooper, B., and Sosna, U. (1980). Family settings of the psychiatrically disturbed aged. In *The social consequences of psychiatric illness* (ed. L.N. Robins, P.J. Clayton, and J.K. Wing), pp. 141–57. Brunner Mazel, New York.

Cooper, B., Harwin, B.G., Depla, C., and Shepherd, M. (1975). Mental health care in the community: an evaluative study. *Psychological Medicine*, **5,** 372–80.

Cooper, J. (1979). Crisis admission units and emergency psychiatric services. *Public Health in Europe*, No. 11. World Health Organization, Copenhagen.

Cooper, J.E. (1980). The description and classification of social disability by means of a taxonomic hierarchy. *Acta Psychiatrica Scandinavica*, **62,** Supplement 285, 140–6.

Cooper, J.E., and Bostock, J. (1988). Relationships between schizophrenia, social disability, symptoms and diagnosis. In *Handbook of social psychiatry* (ed. A.S. Henderson and G.D. Burrows). Elsevier, Amsterdam.

Cooper, J., and Sartorius, N. (1977). Cultural and temporal variations in schizophrenia: a speculation on the importance of industrialization. *British Journal of Psychiatry*, **130,** 50–5.

Copeland, J.R.M. (1981). Mental illness amongst the elderly in London. In: *Epidemiology and prevention of mental illness in old age*. (ed. E. Magnussen, J. Nielsen and J. Buch), pp. 63–6. Nordisk Samrad for Eldreaktivitet, Hellerup.

Copeland, J.R.M., Dewey, M., and Griffiths-Jones, H. (1986*a*). A standardised assessment of mental state and diagnosis in the elderly: GMS and AGECAT. In *Psychiatric disorders in the elderly* (ed. P.E. Bebbington and R. Jacoby). Mental Health Foundation, London.

Copeland, J.R.M., Dewey, M.E., and Griffiths-Jones, H.M. (1986*b*). Computerised psychiatric diagnostic system and case nomenclature for elderly persons. GMS and AGECAT. *Psychological Medicine*, **16,** 89–99.

Copeland, J.R.M., Gurland, B.J., Dewey, M.E., Kelleher, M.J., Smith, A.M.R., and Davidson, I.A. (1987). Is there more dementia, depression and neurosis in New York? A comparative community study of the elderly in New York and London, using the computer diagnosis, AGECAT. *British Journal of Psychiatry*, **151,** 466–73.

Copeland, J.R.M. *et al.* (1976). A semi-structured clinical interview for the assessment of diagnosis and mental state in the elderly: the Geriatric Mental State Schedule. I. Development and reliability. *Psychological Medicine*, **6,** 439–49.

Copeland, J.R.M. *et al.* (1988). The Geriatric Mental State and AGECAT diagnosis in community studies. *Psychological Medicine*, **8,** 219–23.

Corney, R.H. (1982). The effectiveness of social work intervention in the management of depressed women in general practice. In *Social work and primary health care* (ed. A.W. Clare and R.H. Corney). Academic Press, London.

Corney, R.H. (1984). The mental and physical health of clients referred to social workers in a local authority department and a general practice attachment scheme. *Psychological Medicine*, **14,** 137–44.

Corney, R.H. (1985). Social work in general practice. *Journal of the Royal College of General Practitioners*, **35,** 291–2.

Cox, J.L. (ed.) (1986). *Transcultural psychiatry*. Croom Helm, London.

Crawford, A., Plant, M., Kreitman, N., and Latcham, R. (1984). Regional variations in British alcohol morbidity rates: a myth uncovered? II. Population surveys. *British Medical Journal*, **289,** 134–5.

Crawford, A., Plant, M., Kreitman, N., and Latcham, R. (1985). Self-reported alcohol consumption and adverse consequences of drinking in three areas of Britain: general population studies. *British Journal of Addiction*, **80,** 421–8.

Creer, C., and Wing, J.K. (1974). *Schizophrenia at home*. National Schizophrenia Fellowship, London.

Crocetti, G.M., Lemkau, P.V., Kulcar, Z., and Kesic, B. (1971). Selected aspects of the epidemiology of psychoses in Croatia, Yugoslavia. III. The cluster sample and the results of the pilot survey. *American Journal of Epidemiology*, **94,** 126–34.

Davenport, S., Goldberg, D., and Millar, T. (1987). How psychiatric disorders are missed during medical consultations. *Lancet*, **2,** 439–40.

Day, R. *et al.* (1987). Stressful life events preceding the acute onset of schizophrenia: a cross-national study from the World Health Organization. *Culture, Medicine and Psychiatry*, **11,** 123–205.

De Jong, A., Giel, R., Sloof, C.J., and Wiersma, D. (1985). Social disability and outcome in schizophrenic patients. *British Journal of Psychiatry*, **147,** 631–6.

Der, G., and Bebbington, P.E. (1987). Depression in inner London: a register study. *Social Psychiatry*, **22,** 73–84.

Derogatis, L.R., Rickels, K., Uhlenhuth, E.H., and Covi, L. (1974). The Hopkins Symptoms Checklist (HSCL): a measure of primary symptom dimensions. In *Psychological measurements in psychopharmacology. Modern problems for the pharmacopsychiatrist* (ed. P. Pichot), Vol. 7, pp. 70–110. Karger, Basel.

Diener, E. (1984). Subjective well-being. *Psychological Bulletin*, **95,** 542–75.

Dohrenwend, B.P., and Dohrenwend, B.S. (1969). *Social status and psychological disorder: A causal inquiry*, pp. 9–31. Wiley-Interscience, New York.

Dohrenwend, B.P., and Dohrenwend, B.S. (1980). Psychiatric disorders and susceptibility to stress. In *The social consequences of psychiatric illness* (ed. L.N. Robins, P.J. Clayton, and J.K. Wing, pp. 183–97. Brunner Mazel, New York.

Dohrenwend, B.P., and Dohrenwend, B.S. (1981). Socioenvironmental factors, stress and psychopathology. *American Journal of Community Psychology*, **9,** 124–64.

Drew, L.R.H. (1968). Alcoholism as a self-limiting disease. *Australian Journal of Alcohol Studies*, **29,** 956–67.

Duncan-Jones, P. (1981*a*). The structure of social relationships: analysis of a survey instrument. 1. *Social Psychiatry*, **16,** 55–61.

Duncan-Jones, P. (1981*b*). The structure of social relationships: analysis of a survey instrument. 2. *Social Psychiatry*, **16,** 143–9.

Duncan-Jones, P., and Henderson, S. (1978). The use of a two-phase design in a population survey. *Social Psychiatry*, **13,** 231–7.

Duncan-Jones, P., Grayson, D.A., and Moran, P.A.P. (1986). The utility of latent trait models in psychiatric epidemiology. *Psychological Medicine*, **16,** 391–405.

Dupont, A. (1980). A study concerning the time-related and other burdens when severely handicapped children are reared at home. *Acta Psychiatrica Scandinavica*, **285,** 249–57.

Dupont A. (1986). Socio-psychiatric aspects of the young severely mentally retarded and family. *British Journal of Psychiatry*, **148,** 227–34.

Durkheim, E. (1897). *Le suicide: Etude de sociologie*. Felix Alcan, Paris.

Earll, L., and Kincey, J. (1982). Clinical psychology in general practice. A controlled trial evaluation. *Journal of the Royal College of General Practitioners*, **32,** 32–7.

Eastman, C., and McPherson, I. (1982). As others see us: GPs' perceptions of psychological problems and the relevance of clinical psychology. *British Journal of Clinical Psychology*, **21,** 85–92.

Eastwood, M.R. (1975). *The relation between physical and mental illness*. University of Toronto Press.

Eaton, W.W. (1975). Causal models for the study of prevalence. *Social Forces*, **34,** 415–426.

Eaton, W.W. (1980). *The sociology of mental disorders*. Praeger, New York.

Eaton, W.W. (1985). Epidemiology of schizophrenia. *Epidemiologic Review*, **7,** 105–26.

Edwards, G. (1980). Epidemiology applied to alcoholism. In: *Alcoholism. Introduction to theory and treatment* (ed. D.A. Ward), pp. 82–100. Kendall-Hunt, Iowa.

Edwards, G., and Gross, M.M. (1976). Alcohol dependence: provisional description of a clinical syndrome. *British Journal of Medicine*, **1,** 1058–61.

Eisenberg, L. (1987). Preventing mental, neurological and psychosocial disorders. *World Health Forum*, **8,** 245–53.

Eisenberg, P., and Lazarsfeld, P.F. (1938). The psychological effects of unemployment. *Psychological Bulletin*, **35,** 358–90.

Eitinger, L. (1964). *Concentration camp survivors in Norway and Israel*. Oslo University Press, Oslo.

Endicott, J., and Spitzer, R.L. (1978). A diagnostic interview. *Archives of General Psychiatry*, **35,** 837–44.

Esquirol, J.E. (1967). A treatise on insanity [1845]. In *Documentary history of psychiatry. A source book on historical principles* (ed. C.E. Goshen), pp. 314–69. Philosophical Library, New York.

Essen-Möller, E. (1956). Individual traits and morbidity in a Swedish rural population. *Acta Psychiatrica Scandinavica*, Supplement 100, 5–160.

Essex, B., and Gosling, H. (1983). An algorithmic method for management of mental health problems in developing countries. *British Journal of Psychiatry*, **143,** 451–9.

Eysenck, H.J., and Eysenck, S.B.G. (1964). *Manual of the Eysenck Personality Inventory*. London University Press, London.

Fadden, G., Bebbington, P., and Kuipers, L. (1987*a*). The burden of care:

the impact of functional psychiatric illness on the patient's family. *British Journal of Psychiatry*, **150,** 285–92.

Fadden, G.B., Bebbington P., and Kuipers, L. (1987*b*). Caring and its burdens: a study of the spouses of depressed patients. *British Journal of Psychiatry*, **151,** 660–7.

Falloon, R.H., and Liberman, R.P. (1983). Interactions between drug and psychosocial therapy in schizophrenia. *Schizophrenia Bulletin*, **9,** 543–54.

Farber, B.A. (ed.) (1983). *Stress and burnout in the human service professions*. Pergamon Press, New York.

Faris, E. (1932). The primary group: essence and accident. *American Journal of Sociology*, **38,** 41–50.

Faris, R.E.L., and Dunham, H.W. (1939). *Mental disorders in urban areas*. University of Chicago Press.

Faris, R.E.L., and Dunham, H.W. (1960). *Mental disorders in urban areas. An ecological study of schizophrenia and other psychoses*. Hafner, New York.

Feather, N.I., and Barber, J.G. (1983). Depressive reactions and unemployment. *Journal of Abnormal Psychology*, **92,** 185–95.

Fergusson, D.M., Horwood, L.J., and Lawton, J.M. (in press). The relationships between neuroticism and depressive symptoms. *Social Psychiatry*.

Finlay-Jones, R.A. (1988). Life events and psychiatric illness. In *Handbook of social psychiatry*. (ed. A.S. Henderson and G.D. Burrows). Elsevier, Amsterdam.

Finlay-Jones, R., and Brown, G.W. (1981). Types of stressful life events and the onset of anxiety and depressive disorders. *Psychological Medicine*, **11,** 803–15.

Finlay-Jones, R., and Eckhardt, B. (1984). A social and psychiatric survey of unemployment among young people. *Australian and New Zealand Journal of Psychiatry*, **18,** 135–43.

Flaherty, J.A., Gaviria, F.M., and Pathak, D.S. (1983). The measurement of social support: the Social Support Network Inventory. *Comprehensive Psychiatry*, **24,** 521–9.

Folstein, M.F., Folstein, S.E., and McHugh, P.R. (1975). 'Mini-Mental State': a practical method for grading the cognitive state of patients for the clinician. *Journal of Psychiatric Research*, **12,** 189–98.

Folstein, M., Anthony, J.C., Parhad, I., Duffy, B., and Gruenberg, E.M. (1985). The meaning of cognitive impairment in the elderly. *Journal of the American Geriatric Society*, **33,** 228–35.

Foulds, G.A. (1965). *Personality and personal illness*. Tavistock, London.

Frank, J.D. (1973). *Persuasion and healing*. Johns Hopkins University Press, Baltimore.

Frank, J.D. (1974). Psychotherapy: the restoration of morale. *American Journal of Psychiatry*, **131,** 271–4.

Frank, J.D. (1977). The two faces of psychotherapy. *Journal of Nervous and Mental Disease*, **164,** 3–7.

Frank, J.D. (1986). What is psychotherapy? In *An introduction to the psychotherapies* (ed. S. Bloch), pp 1–23. Oxford University Press.

Freeman, D. (1983). *Margaret Mead and Samoa. The making and unmaking of an anthropological myth.* Australian National University Press; Canberra.

Fremming, K.H. (1947). The expectancy of mental disorders. *Acta Psychiatrica et Neurologica Scandinavica*, Supplement 52.

Gask, L., McGrath, G., Goldberg, D., and Millar, T. (1987). Improving the psychiatric skills of established general practitioners: evaluation of group teaching. *Medical Education*, **21,** 362–8.

Gask, L., Goldberg, D., Lesser, A.L., and Millar T. (1988). Improving the psychiatric skills of the general practice trainee: an evaluation of a group training course. *Medical Education*, **22,** 132–8.

Gavrilova, S. (1984). Demonstrability of mental disorders in late middle and old age. (Russian). *Zhurnal Nevropatologii i Psikhiatrii*, **84,** 911–18.

Gershon, E.S., and Guroff, J.J. (1984). Information from relatives. *Archives of General Psychiatry*, **41,** 173–80.

Gibbons, J.S., Butler, J., Urwin, P., and Gibbons, J.L. (1978). Evaluation of a social work service for self-poisoning patients. *British Journal of Psychiatry*, **133,** 111–18.

Giel, R. *et al.* (1981). Childhood mental disorders in primary health care: results of observations in four developing countries. *Pediatrics*, **68,** 677–83.

Giel, R. *et al.* (1983). The burden of mental illness on the family. *Acta Psychiatrica Scandinavica*, **68,** 186–201.

Giel, R. *et al.* (1988). The detection of childhood mental disorders in primary care in some developing countries. In *Handbook of social psychiatry* (ed. A.S. Henderson and G.D. Burrows). Elsevier, Amsterdam.

Glass, N.J., and Goldberg, D. (1977). Cost–benefit analysis and the evaluation of psychiatric services. *Psychological Medicine*, **7,** 701–7.

Goldberg, D.P. (1972). *The detection of psychiatric illness by questionnaire.* Maudsley Monographs No. 21. Oxford University Press.

Goldberg, D. (1978). *Manual of the General Health Questionnaire.* NFER Publishing, Windsor.

Goldberg, D. (1982). The concept of a psychiatric 'case' in general practice. *Social Psychiatry*, **17,** 61–5.

Goldberg, D. (1985). Identifying psychiatric illness among general medical patients. *British Medical Journal* **291,** 161–2.

Goldberg, D.P., and Blackwell, B. (1970). Psychiatric illness in general practice. A detailed study using a method of case identification. *British Medical Journal*, **2,** 439–43.

Goldberg, D.P., and Hillier, V.F. (1979). A scaled version of the General Health Questionnaire. *Psychological Medicine*, **9,** 139–45.

Goldberg, D.P., and Huxley, P. (1980). *Mental illness in the community: The pathway to psychiatric care*. Tavistock, London.

Goldberg, D., and Jones, R. (1980). The costs and benefits of psychiatric care. In *The social consequences of psychiatric illness* (ed. L. Robins, P. Clayton, and J. Wing), pp. 55–70. Brunner-Mazel, New York.

Goldberg, D.P., and Williams, P. (1988). *A user's guide to the GHQ*. NFER Nelson, London.

Goldberg, D.P., Cooper, B., Eastwood, M.R., Kedward, H.B., and Shepherd, M. (1970). A standardized psychiatric interview for use in community surveys. *British Journal of Preventive and Social Medicine*, **24,** 18–23.

Goldberg, D.P., Steele, J.J., Smith, C., and Spivey, L. (1980). Training family doctors to recognize psychiatric illness with increased accuracy. *Lancet*, **2,** 521–3.

Goldberg, D.P., Bridges, K., Duncan-Jones, P., and Grayson, D. (1987). Dimensions of neuroses seen in primary care settings. *Psychological Medicine*, **17,** 461–70.

Goldberg, E.M., and Morrison, S.L. (1963). Schizophrenia and social class. *British Journal of Psychiatry*, **109,** 785–802.

Goldhamer, H., and Marshall, A.W. (1953). *Psychosis and civilization: Two studies in the frequency of mental disease*. The Free Press, Glencoe, Illinois.

Goodchild, M.E., and Duncan-Jones, P. (1985). Chronicity and the General Health Questionnaire. *British Journal of Psychiatry*, **146,** 55–61.

Grad, J., and Sainsbury, P. (1966*a*). The evaluations: evaluating the community psychiatric service in Chichester: aims and methods of research. *Milbank Memorial Fund Quarterly*, **44,** Part 2, 231–42.

Grad, J., and Sainsbury, P. (1966*b*). The evaluations: evaluating the community psychiatric service in Chichester: results. *Milbank Memorial Fund Quarterly*, **44,** Part 2, 246–90.

Grad, J., and Sainsbury, P. (1968). The effects that patients have on their families in a community care and a control psychiatric service—a two-year follow-up study. *British Journal of Psychiatry*, **114,** 265–78.

Graham, P.J. (ed) (1977). *Epidemiological approaches in child psychiatry*. Academic Press, London.

Grayson, D.A., Henderson, A.S., and Kay, D.W.K. (1987). Diagnoses of dementia and depression: a latent trait analysis of their performance. *Psychological Medicine*, **17,** 667–75.

Greenblatt, M., Becerra, R.M., and Serafetinides, E.A. (1982). Social networks and mental health: an overview. *American Journal of Psychiatry*, **139,** 977–84.

Greenwood, M. (1935). *Epidemic and crowd diseases*. Williams and Norgate, London.

Gruenberg, E. (1974). The social breakdown syndrome and its prevention. In

American handbook of psychiatry. Vol. 2: *Child and adolescent psychiatry, sociocultural and community psychiatry* (ed. G. Caplan), pp. 697–711. Basic Books, New York.

Gruenberg, E.M. (1977). The failures of success. *Milbank Memorial Fund Quarterly*, **55,** 3–24.

Gruenberg, E.M., and Kennedy, C. (1988). Some determinants of chronic disability. In *Handbook of social psychiatry* (ed. A.S. Henderson and G.D. Burrows). Elsevier, Amsterdam.

Gruenberg, E.M., Hagnell, O., Ojesjo, L., and Mittelman, M. (1976). *The rising prevalence of chronic brain syndrome in the elderly*. Paper presented at the Symposium on Society, Stress and Disease: Aging and Old Age, Stockholm, 14–19 June.

Gunderson, J.G., and Mosher, L.R. (1975). The cost of schizophrenia. *American Journal of Psychiatry*, **132,** 901–6.

Gunn, J. (1979). Forensic psychiatry. In *Recent advances in clinical psychiatry* (ed. K. Granville-Grossman), pp. 271–95. Churchill Livingstone, Edinburgh.

Gunn, J. (1982). Forensic psychiatry as a subspecialty. *International Journal of Law and Psychiatry*, **5,** 65–79.

Gunn, J. (1986). Education and forensic psychiatry. *Canadian Journal of Psychiatry*, **31,** 273–80.

Gurland, B., Copeland, J., Kuriansky, J., Kelleher, M., Sharpe, L., and Dean, L. (1983). *The mind and mood of aging*. Croom Helm, London.

Häfner, H. (1985). Are mental disorders increasing over time? *Psychopathology*, **18,** 66–81.

Hagnell, O. (1966). *A prospective study of the incidence of mental disorder*. Scandinavian University Books, Svenska Bokforlaget, Norstedts-Bonniers, Stockholm.

Hagnell, O. (1981). The Lundby Study on Psychiatric Morbidity (Sweden). In *Prospective longitudinal research: An empirical basis for the primary prevention of psychosocial disorders* (ed. S.A. Mednick, and A.E. Baert), pp. 189–206. Oxford University Press.

Hagnell, O., Nyman, E., and Tinving, K. (1973). Dangerous alcoholics. Personality varieties in aggressive and suicidally inclined subjects. *Scandinavian Journal of Social Medicine*, **3,** 125–31.

Hagnell, O., Lanke, J., Rorsman, B., and Ojesjo, L. (1981). Does the incidence of age psychosis decrease? A prospective longitudinal study of a complete population investigated during the 25-year period 1947–1972: the Lundby Study. *Neuropsychobiology*, **7,** 201–11.

Hagnell, O., Lanke, J., Rorsman, B., and Ojesjo, L. (1982). Are we entering an age of melancholy? Depressive illnesses in a prospective epidemiological study over 25 years: the Lundby Study, Sweden. *Psychological Medicine*, **12,** 279–89.

Hagnell, O., Lanke, J., Rorsman, B., Ohman, R., and Ojesjo, L. (1983). Current trends in the incidence of senile and multi-infarct dementia. *Archives of Psychiatry and Neurological Sciences*, **233,** 423–38.

Haley, J. (1971). *Changing families: A family therapy reader*. Grune & Stratton, New York.

Haley, J. (1977). *Problem solving therapy*. Bassey-Joss, San Francisco.

Hamburg, D.A. (1968*a*). Emotions in the perspective of human evolution. In *Perspectives on human evolution*, Vol. 1 (eds S.L. Washburn and P.C. Jay), pp. 246–57. Holt, Rinehart & Winston, New York.

Hamburg, D.A. (1968*b*). Evolution of emotional responses: evidence from recent research on nonhuman primates. *Science and Psychoanalysis*, **12,** 39–54.

Harding, T.W. *et al.* (1983*a*). The World Health Organization Collaborative Study on Strategies for Extending Mental Health Care. II. The development of new research methods. *American Journal of Psychiatry*, **140,** 1474–80.

Harding, T.W. *et al.* (1983*b*). The World Health Organization Collaborative Study on Strategies for Extending Mental Health Care. III. Evaluative design and illustrative results. *American Journal of Psychiatry*, **140,** 1481–5.

Hare, E. (1983). Was insanity on the increase? *British Journal of Psychiatry*, **142,** 439–55.

Hare, E.H. (1987). Epidemiology of schizophrenia and affective psychoses. *British Medical Bulletin*, **43,** 514–30.

Hare, E.H., and Shaw, G.K. (1965). *Mental health on a new housing estate*. Maudsley Monographs, No. 12. Oxford University Press.

Harris, T. (1988). Psychosocial vulnerability to depression: the biographical perspective of the Bedford College studies. In *Handbook of social psychiatry* (ed. A.S. Henderson and G.D. Burrows). Elsevier, Amsterdam.

Harris, T., Brown, G.W., and Bifulco, A. (1986). Loss of parent in childhood and adult psychiatric disorder: the role of lack of adequate parental care. *Psychological Medicine*, **16,** 641–59.

Harris, T., Brown, G.W., and Bifulco, A. (1987). Loss of parent in childhood and adult psychiatric disorder: the role of social class position and premarital pregnancy. *Psychological Medicine*, **17,** 163–83.

Hasegawa, K. (1979). Aspects of community mental health care of the elderly in Japan. *International Journal of Mental Health*, **8,** 36–49.

Hasegawa, K. *et al.* (1984). The prevalence study of age-related dementia in the community. (*Japanese*) *Geriatric Psychiatry*, **1,** 94–105.

Helgason, T. (1964). Epidemiology of mental disorders in Iceland. *Acta Psychiatrica Scandinavica*, **40,** Supplement 173, 1–258.

Helzer, J.E. (1981). Methodological issues in the interpretations of the consequences of extreme situations. In *Stressful life events and their contexts* (B.S. Dohrenwend and B.P. Dohrenwend), pp. 108–29. Prodist, New York.

Helzer, J.E., Robins, L.N., Wish, E., and Hesselbrock, M. (1979). Depression in Vietnam veterans and civilian controls. *American Journal of Psychiatry*, **136,** 526–9.

Henderson, A.S. (1974). Care-eliciting behavior in man. *Journal of Nervous and Mental Disease*, **159,** 172–81.

Henderson, S. (1980). Personal networks and the schizophrenias. *Australian and New Zealand Journal of Psychiatry*, **14,** 255–9.

Henderson, A.S. (1984). Interpreting the evidence on social support. *Social Psychiatry*, **19,** 49–52.

Henderson, A.S. (1985). Methods of data collection and analysis as a prerequisite for progress in classification. In *Mental disorders, alcohol- and drug-related problems. International perspectives on their diagnosis and classification*, pp. 151–8. Excerpta Medica, Amsterdam.

Henderson, A.S. (1986). The epidemiology of Alzheimer's disease. *British Medical Bulletin*, **42,** 3–10.

Henderson, A.S., and Bostock, F.T. (1975). Coping behaviour: correlates of survival on a raft. *Australian and New Zealand Journal of Psychiatry*, **9,** 221–3.

Henderson, S., and Bostock, T. (1977). Coping behaviour after shipwreck. *British Journal of Psychiatry*, **131,** 15–20.

Henderson, A.S., and Brown, G.W. (1988). Social support: the hypothesis and the evidence. In *Handbook of social psychiatry* (ed. A.S. Henderson and G.D. Burrows). Elsevier, Amsterdam.

Henderson, A.S., and Huppert, F.A. (1984). The problem of mild dementia. *Psychological Medicine*, **14,** 5–11.

Henderson, S., Byrne, D.G., Duncan-Jones, P., Adcock, S., Scott, R., and Steele, G.P. (1978*a*). Social bonds in the epidemiology of neurosis: a preliminary communication. *British Journal of Psychiatry*, **132,** 463–6.

Henderson, S., Duncan-Jones, P., McAuley, H., and Ritchie, K. (1978*b*). The patient's primary group. *British Journal of Psychiatry*, **132,** 74–86.

Henderson, S., Duncan-Jones, P., Byrne, D.G., and Scott, R. (1980). Measuring social relationships: the Interview Schedule for Social Interaction. *Psychological Medicine*, **10,** 723–34.

Henderson, S. with Byrne, D.G., and Duncan-Jones, P. (1981). *Neurosis and the social environment*. Academic Press, Sydney.

Henderson, A.S., Grayson, D.A., Scott, R., Wilson, J., Rickwood, D., and Kay, D.W.K. (1986*a*). Social support, dementia and depression among the elderly living in the Hobart community. *Psychological Medicine*, **16,** 379–90.

Henderson, A.S., Scott, R., and Kay, D.W.K. (1986*b*). The elderly who live alone: their mental health and social relationships. *Australian and New Zealand Journal of Psychiatry*, **20,** 202–9.

Hinkle, L.E., and Wolff, H.G. (1957*a*). The nature of man's adaptation to his total environment and the relation of this to illness. *Archives of Internal Medicine*, **99,** 442–60.

Hinkle, L.E., and Wolff, H.G. (1957*b*). Health and the social environment: experimental investigations. In *Explorations in social psychiatry* (ed. A.H. Leighton, J.A. Clausen, and R.N. Wilson), pp. 105–37. Basic Books, New York.

Hoeper, E.W., Nycz, G.R., Kessler, L.G., Burke, J.D., and Pierce, W.E. (1984). The usefulness of screening for mental illness. *Lancet*, **1,** 33–5.

Holmes, T.H., and Rahe, R.H. (1967). The Social Readjustment Rating Scale. *Journal of Psychosomatic Research*, **11,** 213–18.

Hooley, J.M. (1986). II. Family attributes. 2. An introduction to EE measurement and research. In *Treatment of schizophrenia. Family assessment and intervention* (ed. M.J. Goldstein, I. Hand, and K. Hahlweg). Springer-Verlag, Berlin.

Hoult, J., Reynolds, I., Charbonneau-Powis, M., Coles, P., and Briggs, J. (1981). A controlled study of psychiatric hospital versus community treatment—the effect on relatives. *Australian and New Zealand Journal of Psychiatry*, **15,** 323–8.

Hoult, J., Rosen, A., and Reynolds, I. (1984). Community orientated treatment compared to psychiatric hospital orientated treatment. *Social Science and Medicine*, **18,** 1005–10.

Ibrahim, M.A., and Spitzer, W.O. (1979). The case-control study: the problem and the prospect. *Journal of Chronic Diseases*, **32,** 139–44.

Ignacio, L.L. *et al.* (1983). Knowledge and attitudes of primary health care personnel concerning mental health problems in developing countries. *American Journal of Public Health*, **73,** 1081–4.

Ingham, J.G., and Miller, P.M. (1976). The concept of prevalence applied to psychiatric disorders and symptoms. *Psychological Medicine*, **6,** 217–25.

Ingham, J., and Miller, P. (1982). Consulting with mild symptoms in general practice. *Social Psychiatry*, **17,** 77–88.

Iwanicki, E.F., and Schwab, R.L. (1981). A cross-validation study of the Maslach Burnout Inventory. *Educational and Psychological Measurement*, **41,** 1167–74.

Jablensky, A. (1985). Objectives and progress of the WHO/ADMAHA Joint Project and Classification of Mental Disorders and Alcohol- and Drug-related Problems. In *Mental disorders; Alcohol- and drug-related problems. International perspectives on their diagnosis and classification*, pp. 74–9. Excerpta Medica: Amsterdam.

Jablensky, A., Schwarz, R., and Tomov, T. (1980). World Health Organization collaborative study on impairments and disabilities associated with

Schizophrenic Disorders. *Acta Psychiatrica Scandinavica*, **62,** Supplement 285, 152–63.

Jackson, P.R., and Warr, P. (1987). Mental health of unemployed men in different parts of England and Wales. *British Medical Journal*, **295,** 525.

Jacobson, S., Fasman, J., and DiMascio, A. (1975). Deprivation in the childhood of depressed women. *Journal of Nervous and Mental Disease*, **160,** 4–13.

Jarvik, L.F., Ruth, V., and Matsuyama, S.S. (1980). Organic brain syndrome and aging: a six-year follow-up of surviving twins. *Archives of General Psychiatry*, **37,** 280–6.

Jaspers, K. (1962). *General psychopathology*, 7th edn (trans. J. Hoenig and M.W. Hamilton). Manchester University Press.

Jencks, S.F. (1985). Recognition of mental distress and diagnosis of mental disorder in primary care. *Journal of the American Medical Association*, **253,** 1903–7.

Jenkins, R. (1985). Sex differences in minor psychiatric morbidity. *Psychological Medicine*, Supplement No. 7, 1–53.

Jenkins, J., Felce, D., Lunt, B., and Powell, L. (1977). Increasing engagement in activity of residents in old people's homes by providing recreational materials. *Behaviour Research and Therapy*, **15,** 429–34.

Jennings, C., Barraclough, B.M., and Moss, J.R. (1987). Have the Samaritans lowered the suicide rate? A controlled study. *Psychological Medicine*, **8,** 413–33.

Jensen, K. (1963). Psychiatric problems in four Danish old age homes. *Acta Psychiatrica Scandinavica*, Supplement, **169,** 411–19.

Jeste, D.V., Carmen, R., Lohr, J.B., and Wyatt, R.J. (1985). Did schizophrenia exist before the eighteenth century? *Comprehensive Psychiatry*, **26,** 493–503.

Johnstone, A., and Goldberg, D. (1976). Psychiatric screening in general practice: a controlled trial. *Lancet*, **1,** 605–8.

Jorm, A.F. (1987). *Modifiability of a personality trait which is a risk factor for neurosis*. Paper presented to the World Psychiatric Association Symposium on Epidemiology and the Prevention of Mental Disorder, Reykavik, 15–17 September.

Jorm, A.F., Korten, A., and Henderson, A.S. (1987). The prevalence of dementia: a quantitative integration of the literature. *Acta Psychiatrica Scandinavica*, **76,** 465–79.

Kahn, R.L., and Antonucci, T.C. (1980). Convoys over the life course: attachment, roles and social support. *Life Span Development and Behavior*, **3,** 253–86.

Kahn, R.L., Goldfarb, A.I., Pollack, M., and Peck, A. (1960). Brief objective measures for the determination of mental status in the aged. *American Journal of Psychiatry*, **117,** 326–8.

Kaneko, Z. (1975). Care in Japan. In *Modern perspectives in the psychiatry of old age* (ed. J.G. Howells), pp. 519–30. Brunner Mazel, New York.

Karasawa, A., Kawashima, K., and Kasahara, H. (1982). *Epidemiological study of the senile in Tokyo metropolitan area*, pp. 285–9. Proceedings of World Psychiatric Association Regional Symposium.

Karno, M. *et al.* (1987). Expressed emotion and schizophrenic outcome among Mexican–American families. *Journal of Nervous and Mental Disease*, **175,** 143–51.

Katz, R., and McGuffin, P. (1987). Neuroticism in familial depression. *Psychological Medicine*, **17,** 155–61.

Kay, D.W.K., Beamish, P., and Roth, M. (1964). Old age mental disorders in Newcastle upon Tyne. Part I. A study of prevalence. *British Journal of Psychiatry*, **110,** 146–58.

Kay, D.W.K., Henderson, A.S., Scott, R., Wilson, J., Rickwood, D., and Grayson, D.A. (1985). Dementia and depression among the elderly living in the Hobart community: the effect of the diagnostic criteria on the prevalence rates. *Psychological Medicine*, **15,** 771–88.

Kelleher, M.J., and Copeland, J.R. (1973). Psychiatric diagnosis in Cork and London: results of a cross-national pilot study. *Journal of the Irish Medical Association*, **66,** 553–5.

Kelleher, M.J., and Copeland, J.R. (1974). Psychiatric diagnosis in Ireland: a videotape study. *Journal of the Irish Medical Association*, **67,** 87–92.

Kendell, R.E. (1975). *The role of diagnosis in psychiatry*. Blackwell, Oxford.

Kendell, R.E., Hall, D.J., Hailey, A., and Babigian, H.M. (1973). The epidemiology of anorexia nervosa. *Psychological Medicine*, **3,** 200–3.

Kennedy, P.F., and Kreitman, N. (1973). An epidemiological survey of parasuicide ('attempted suicide') in general practice. *British Journal of Psychiatry*, **123,** 23–34.

Kessel, W.I.N. (1960). Psychiatric morbidity in a London general practice. *British Journal of Preventive and Social Medicine*, **14,** 16–22.

Kessler, L.G., Cleary, P.D., and Burke, J.D. (1985). Psychiatric disorders in primary care. *Archives of General Psychiatry*, **42,** 583–7.

Kiev, A. (1972). *Transcultural psychiatry*. Free Press, New York.

Kiff, J. (1981). *Stress, personality and illness*. Unpublished D.Phil. thesis. University of Edinburgh.

Kleinman, A. (1986). *Social origins of distress and disease*. Yale University Press, New Haven and London.

Kleinman, A., and Kleinman, J. (1985). Somatization. The interconnections among culture, depressive experiences and the meaning of pain. In *Culture and depression*. (ed. A. Kleinman and B. Good). University of California Press, Los Angeles.

Klerman, G.L. (1987). *The current age of youthful melancholia: evidence for increase in depression among adolescents and young adults*. 3rd Eli Lilly Lecture, Meeting of the Royal College of Psychiatrists, January 1987.

Klerman, G.L., and Izen, J.E. (1977). The effect of bereavement and grief on physical health and general well-being. *Advances in Psychosomatic Medicine*, **9,** 63–104.

Klerman, G.L., Lavori, P., Rice, J., and Reich, T. (1985). Birth-cohort trends in rates of major depressive disorder among relatives of patients with affective disorder. *Archives of General Psychiatry*, **42,** 689–93.

Kramer, M. (1983). The increasing prevalence of mental disorder: a pandemic threat. *Psychiatric Quarterly*, **55,** 115–43.

Kramer, M., German, P.S., Anthony, J.C., Von Korff, M., and Skinner, E.A. (1985). Patterns of mental disorders among the elderly residents of eastern Baltimore. *Journal of the American Geriatric Society*, **33,** 236–45.

Kraus, A.S., and Lilienfeld, A.M. (1959). Some epidemiologic aspects of the high mortality rate in the young widowed group. *Journal of Chronic Disease*, **10,** 207–17.

Kreitman, N. (1961). The reliability of psychiatric diagnosis. *Journal of Mental Science*, **107,** 876–86.

Kreitman, N. (1964). The patient's spouse. *British Journal of Psychiatry*, **110,** 159–73.

Kreitman, N. (1977*a*). Three themes in the epidemiology of alcoholism. In *Alcoholism. New knowledge and new responses* (ed. G. Edwards and M. Grant), pp. 48–59. Croom Helm, London.

Kreitman, N. (ed.) (1977*b*). *Parasuicide*. Wiley, London.

Kreitman, N. (1980). Introduction to the consequences of psychiatric disorder for life stress and interpersonal relationships. In *The social consequences of psychiatric illness* (ed. L.N. Robins, P.J. Clayton, and J.K. Wing), pp. 135–40. Brunner Mazel, New York.

Kreitman, N. (1986). Alcohol consumption and the preventive paradox. *British Journal of Addiction*, **81,** 353–63.

Kreitman, N. (1988). Suicide and parasuicide. In *Edinburgh companion to psychiatric studies*, 4th edn (ed. A.K. Zealley and R.F. Kendell). Churchill Livingstone, Edinburgh.

Kreitman, N., Pearce, K.I., and Ryle, A. (1966). The relationship of psychiatric, psychosomatic and organic illness in a general practice. *British Journal of Psychiatry*, **112,** 569–79.

Kreitman, N., Collins, J., Nelson, B., and Troop, J. (1970). Neurosis and marital interaction. I. Personality and symptoms. *British Journal of Psychiatry*, **117,** 33–46.

Krupinski, J. (1967). Sociological aspects of health in migrants. *Social Science and Medicine*, **1,** 267–81.

Krupinski, J. (1984). Changing patterns of migration to Australia and their influence on the health of migrants. *Social Science and Medicine*, **18,** 927–37.

Kuipers, L. (1979). Expressed emotion: a review. *British Journal of Social and Clinical Psychology*, **18,** 237–43.

Kuipers, L., and Bebbington, P. (1988). *Living with mental illness*. Souvenir Press, London.

Lambo, T.A. (1966). Psychiatric disorders in the aged: epidemiology and preventative measures. *West African Medical Journal*, **15,** 121–4.

Langer, E.J., and Rodin, J. (1976). The effects of choice and enhanced personal responsibility for the aged: a field experiment in an institutional setting. *Journal of Personality and Social Psychology*, **34,** 191–8.

Lapouse, R., and Monk, M.A. (1958). An epidemiologic study of behaviour characteristics in children. *American Journal of Public Health*, **48,** 1134–44.

Last, J.M. (1983). *A dictionary of epidemiology*. Oxford University Press.

Latcham, R.W., and Kreitman, N. (1984). Regional variation in alcoholism rates in Britain: the effect of provision and use of services. *International Journal of Epidemiology*, **13,** 442–6.

Lazarus, R.S. (1981). The stress and coping paradigm. In *Models for clinical psychopathology* (ed. C. Eisdorfer, D. Cohen, A. Kleinman, and P. Maxim). Medical and Scientific Books, Jamaica.

Leff, J.P. (1981). *Psychiatry around the globe: A transcultural view*. Dekker, New York.

Leff, J., and Vaughn, C. (1980). The interaction of life events and relatives' expressed emotion in schizophrenia and depressive neurosis. *British Journal of Psychiatry*, **136,** 146–53.

Leff, J., and Vaughn, C. (1985). *Expressed emotion in families*. Guildford Press, New York.

Leff, J.P., and Wing, J.K. (1971). Trial of maintenance therapy in schizophrenia. *British Medical Journal*, **3,** 559–604.

Leff, J., Kuipers, L., Berkowitz, R., Ebedein-Vries, R., and Sturgeon, D. (1982). A controlled trial of social intervention in the families of schizophrenic patients. *British Journal of Psychiatry*, **141,** 121–34.

Leff, J., Kuipers, L., Berkowitz, R., Vaughn, C., and Sturgeon, D. (1983). Life events, relatives' expressed emotion and maintenance neuroleptics in schizophrenic relapse. *Psychological Medicine*, **13,** 799–806.

Leff, J. *et al.* (1987). Expressed emotion and schizophrenia in North India. III. Influence of relatives' expressed emotion on the course of schizophrenia in Chandigarh. *British Journal of Psychiatry*, **151,** 166–73.

Leighton, A.H., Lambo, T.A., Hughes, C.C., Leighton, D.C., Murphy, J.M., and Macklin, D.B. (1963). Epidemiology of psychiatric disorder. In *Psychiatric disorder among the Yoruba*, pp. 123–61. Cornell University Press, New York.

Leighton, D.C., Harding, J.S., Macklin, D.B., Macmillan, A.M., and Leighton, A. (1963*a*). *The character of danger*. Basic Books, New York.

Leighton, D.C., Harding, J.S., Macklin, D.B., Hughes, C.C., and Leighton, A.H. (1963*b*). Psychiatric findings of the Stirling County Study. *American Journal of·Psychiatry*, **119,** 1021–6.

Lemkau, P.V., Kulcar, Z., Kesic, B., and Kovacic, L. (1980). Selected aspects of the epidemiology of psychoses in Croatia, Yugoslavia. IV. Representative sample and results of the survey. *American Journal of Epidemiology*, **112,** 661–74.

Lewis, A. (1967). Social psychiatry. In *Inquiries in psychiatry: Clinical and social investigations*, pp. 251–69. Science House, New York.

Lidz, T. (1964). *The family and human adaptation. Three lectures.* Hogarth Press and Institute of Psycho-analysis, London.

Lidz, T., Fleck, S., Cornelison, A., and Terry, D. (1958). The intrafamilial environment of the schizophrenic patient. IV. Parental personalities and family interaction. *American Journal of Orthopsychiatry*, **28,** 764–76.

Lilienfeld, A.M. (1957). Epidemiological methods and inferences in studies of noninfectious diseases. *United States Health Sciences Reports*, **72,** 51–60.

Lilienfeld, A.M., and Lilienfeld, D.E. (1980). *Foundations of epidemiology*, 2nd edn. Oxford University Press, New York.

Lin, T. (1953). A study of the incidence of mental disorder in Chinese and other cultures. *Psychiatry*, **16,** 313–36.

Lindemann, E. (1944). Symptomatology and management of acute grief. *American Journal of Psychiatry*, **101,** 141–8.

Linklater, E. (1934). *Magnus Merriman*. Cape, London.

Links, P.S. (1983). Community surveys of the prevalence of childhood psychiatric disorders: a review. *Child Development*, **54,** 531–48.

Litwak, E., and Szelenyi, I. (1969). Primary group structures and their functions: kin, neighbours and friends. *American Sociological Review*, **34,** 465–81.

Lowenthal, M.F. (1964). Social isolation and mental illness in old age. *American Sociological Review*, **29,** 54–70.

Lowenthal, M.F. (1965). Antecedents of isolation and mental illness in old age. *Archives of General Psychiatry*, **12,** 245–54.

Lucas, R.W., Mullin, P.I., Luna, C.B., and McInroy, D.C. (1977). Psychiatrists and a computer as interrogators of patients with alcohol-related illness: a comparison. *British Journal of Psychiatry*, **131,** 160–7.

Lutz, W. (1986). *Community health surveys: A practical guide for health workers.* Nos 1 to 6. International Epidemiological Association and World Health Organization Regional Offices.

McCallister, L., and Fischer, C.S. (1978). A procedure for surveying personal networks. *Sociological Methods and Research*, **7,** 131–48.

Macdonald, A.J.D. (1986). Do general practitioners 'miss' depression in elderly patients? *British Medical Journal*, **292,** 1365–7.

McFarlane, A. (1985). The effects of stressful life events and disasters: research and theoretical issues. *Australian and New Zealand Journal of Psychiatry*, **19,** 409–21.

McFarlane, A.C. (1986). Post-traumatic morbidity of a disaster: a study of cases presenting for psychiatric treatment. *Journal of Nervous and Mental Disease*, **174,** 4–14.

McFarlane, A.C., and Raphael, B. (1984). Ash Wednesday: the effects of a fire. *Australian and New Zealand Journal of Psychiatry*, **18,** 341–51.

McGuffin, P., Katz, R., and Bebbington, P.E. (1988). The Camberwell Collaborative Depression Study. III. Depression and adversity in the relatives of depressed probands. *British Journal of Psychiatry*, in press.

MacMahon, B., and Pugh, T.F. (1970). *Epidemiology: Principles and methods*. Little, Brown, Boston.

McPherson, I. (1981). Clinical psychology in primary health care. In *Reconstructing psychological practice* (ed. I. McPherson and A. Sutton), pp. 21–41. Croom Helm, London.

McPherson, I., and Sutton, A. (eds) (1981). *Reconstructing psychological practice*. Croom Helm, London.

Maddison, D.C., and Viola, A. (1968). The health of widows in the year following bereavement. *Journal of Psychosomatic Research*, **12,** 297–306.

Mann, A.H., Jenkins, R., and Belsey, E. (1981). The twelve-month outcome of patients with neurotic illness in general practice. *Psychological Medicine*, **11,** 535–50.

Marks, I.M. (1969). *Fears and phobias*. Heinemann, London.

Marks, I. (1981). *Cure and care of neuroses: Theory and practice of behavioral psychotherapy*. Wiley, New York.

Marsella, A.J., Tharp, R.G., and Ciborowski, T.P. (eds) (1979). *Perspectives on cross-cultural psychology*. Academic Press, New York.

Marteau, T.M., and Johnston, M. (1987). Health psychology: the danger of neglecting psychological models. *Bulletin of The British Psychological Society*, **40,** 82–5.

Maslach, C., and Jackson, S.E. (1981). *Maslach Burnout Inventory: Manual*. Consulting Psychologists Press, Palo Alto.

Maslow, A.H. (1968). *Toward a psychology of being*. Van Nostrand, New York.

Matthew, G.K. (1971). Measuring need and evaluating services. In *Portfolio for health problems and progress in medical care* (ed. G. McLachlan), 6th series. Oxford University Press for the Nuffield Provincial Hospitals Trust.

Mechanic, D. (1962). The concept of illness behaviour. *Journal of Chronic Disease*, **15,** 189–94.

Mechanic, D. (1978). *Medical sociology*, 2nd edn. Free Press, New York.

Melin, L., and Götestam, K.G. (1981). The effects of rearranging ward routines on communication and eating behaviors of psychogeriatric patients. *Journal of Applied Behavior Analysis*, **14,** 47–51.

Miller, P.M., and Ingham, J.G. (1976). Friends, confidants and symptoms. *Social Psychiatry*, **11,** 51–8.

Minuchin, S. (1974). *Families and family therapy*. Harvard University Press, Cambridge, Mass.

Minuchin, S. (1984). *Family kaleidoscope*. Harvard University Press, Cambridge, Mass.

Mölsä, P.K., Marttila, R.J., and Rinne, U.K. (1982). Epidemiology of dementia in a Finnish population. *Acta Neurologica Scandinavica*, **65,** 541–52.

Morin, R.C., and Seidman, E. (1986). A social network approach and the revolving door patient. *Schizophrenia Bulletin*, **12,** 262–73.

Mullen, E.J., and Dumpson, J.R. (eds) (1972). *Evaluation of social intervention*. Jossey-Bass, New York.

Murphy, H.B.M. (1982). *Comparative psychiatry. The international and intercultural distribution of mental illness*. Springer-Verlag, New York.

Murray, R.M., Lewis, S.W., and Reverley, A.M. (1985). Towards an aetiological classification of schizophrenia. *Lancet*, **1,** 1023–6.

Murthy, R.S., and Wig, N.N. (1983). The World Health Organization Collaborative Study on Strategies for Extending Mental Health Care, IV: A training approach to enhancing the availability of mental health manpower in a developing country. *American Journal of Psychiatry*, **140,** 1486–90.

Neugebauer, R. (1981). The reliability of life event reports. In *Stressful life events and their contexts* (ed. B.S. Dohrenwend and B.P. Dohrenwend), pp. 85–107. Prodist, New York.

Newcomb, M.D., and Bentler, P.M. (1987). The impact of late adolescent substance use on young adult health status and utilization of health services: a structural-equation model over four years. *Social Science and Medicine*, **24,** 71–82.

Nielsen, J. (1962). Geronto-psychiatric period prevalence investigation in a geographically delimited population. *Acta Psychiatrica Scandinavica*, **38,** 307–30.

Nielsen, J. (1976). The Samsø Project from 1957 to 1974. *Acta Psychiatrica Scandinavica*, **54,** 198–222.

Nuallain, ni M., O'Hare, A., Walsh, D., Blake, B., Halpenny, J.V., and O'Brien, P.F. (1984). The incidence of mental illness in Ireland—patients contacting psychiatric services in three Irish counties. *Irish Journal of Psychiatry*, **Autumn,** 23–29.

Nuckolls, C.B., Cassel, J., and Kaplan, B.H. (1972). Psychosocial assets, life crises and the prognosis of pregnancy. *American Journal of Epidemiology*, **95,** 431–41.

Ødegard, Ø. (1967). Changes in the prognosis of functional psychoses since the days of Kraepelin. *British Journal of Psychiatry*, **113,** 813–22.

Ogden, M. (1983). Psychological assessment by computer. *Lancet*, **1,** 1280.

Parker, G. (1983*a*). *Overprotection: A risk factor in psychosocial development*. Grune & Stratton, New York.

Parker, G. (1983*b*). Parental 'affectionless control' as an antecedent to adult depression. *Archives of General Psychiatry*, **40**, 956–60.

Parker, G. (1984). The measurement of pathogenic parental style and its relevance to psychiatric disorder. *Social Psychiatry*, **19**, 75–81.

Parker, G. (1988). Parental style and parental loss. In *Handbook of social psychiatry* (ed. A.S. Henderson and G.D. Burrows). Elsevier, Amsterdam.

Parker, G., and Barnett, B. (1987). A test of the social support hypothesis. *British Journal of Psychiatry*, **150**, 72–7.

Parker, G., Kiloh, L., and Hayward, L. (1987). Parental representations of neurotic and endogenous depressives. *Journal of Affective Disorders*, **13**, 75–82.

Parkes, C.M. (1970). The first year of bereavement. A longitudinal study of the reaction of London widows to the death of their husbands. *Psychiatry*, **33**, 444–67.

Partridge, E. (1966). *A short etymological dictionary of modern English*. Routledge, London.

Pasamanick, B., and Knobloch, H. (1966). Retrospective studies on the epidemiology of reproductive casualty: old and new. *Merrill-Palmer Quarterly of Behavioral Development*, **12**, 7–26.

Pasamanick, B., Scarpitti, F.R., and Dinitz, S. (1967). *Schizophrenics in the community. An experimental study in the prevention of hospitalisation*. Appleton-Century-Crofts, New York.

Paykel, E.S. (1978). Contribution of life events to causation of psychiatric illness. *Psychological Medicine*, **8**, 245–53.

Paykel, E.S. (1983). Methodological aspects of life events research. *Journal of Psychosomatic Research*, **27**, 341–52.

Paykel, E.S., Prusoff, B.A., and Uhlenhuth, E.H. (1971). Scaling of life events. *Archives of General Psychiatry*, **25**, 340–7.

Perris, H. (1984*a*). Life events and depression: 1. Effect of sex, age and civil status. *Journal of Affective Disorders*, **7**, 11–24.

Perris, H. (1984*b*). Life events and depression: 2. Results in diagnostic subgroups, and in relation to the recurrence of depression. *Journal of Affective Disorders*, **7**, 25–36.

Perris, H. (1984*c*). Life events and depression: 3. Relation to severity of the depressive syndrome. *Journal of Affective Disorders*, **7**, 37–54.

Perris, C., Arrindell, W.A., Perris, H., Eiseman, M., Van Der Ende, J., and Von Knorring, L. (1986). Perceived deprived parental rearing and depression. *British Journal of Psychiatry*, **148**, 170–5.

Perris, C., Jacobsson, L., Lindstrom, H., Von Knorring, L., and Perris, H. (1980). Development of a new inventory for assessing memories of parental rearing behavior. *Acta Psychiatrica Scandinavica*, **61**, 265–74.

Philip, A.E., and McCulloch, J.W. (1966). Use of social indices in psychiatric epidemiology. *British Journal of Preventive and Social Medicine*, **20**, 122–6.

Pilowsky, I. (1969). Abnormal illness behaviour. *British Journal of Medical Psychology*, **42,** 347–51.

Pilowsky, I. (1978). A general classification of abnormal illness behaviours. *British Journal of Medical Psychology*, **51,** 131–7.

Pilowsky, I. (1988). Abnormal illness behaviour. In *Handbook of social psychiatry* (ed. A.S. Henderson and G.D. Burrows). Elsevier, Amsterdam.

Plant, M.A. (1978). Occupation and alcoholism: cause or effect? A controlled study of recruits to the drink trade. *International Journal of Addiction*, **13,** 605–26.

Platt, S. (1985). Measuring the burden of psychiatric illness on the family: an evaluation of some rating scales. *Psychological Medicine*, **15,** 383–93.

Popper, K. (1972). *Objective knowledge. An evolutionary approach.* Oxford University Press.

Power, M.J. (1987). Cognitive theories of depression. In *Theoretical foundations of behavior therapy* (ed. H.J. Eysenck and I. Martin). Plenum, New York.

Power, M.J., and Champion, L.A. (1986). Cognitive approaches to depression: a theoretical critique. *British Journal of Clinical Psychology*, **25,** 201–12.

Primrose, E.J.R. (1962). *Psychological illness: A community study.* Charles C. Thomas, Springfield, Illinois.

Rabkin, J.G., and Streuning, E.L. (1976). Life events, stress and illness. *Science*, **194,** 1013–20.

Raphael, B. (1977). Preventive intervention with the recently bereaved. *Archives of General Psychiatry*, **34,** 1450–4.

Raphael, B. (1983). *The anatomy of bereavement.* Basic Books, New York.

Raphael, B. (1986). *When disaster strikes. A handbook for the caring professions.* Basic Books, New York; Hutchison, London.

Rappaport, J. (1977). *Community psychology: Values, research and action.* Holt, Rinehart and Winston, New York.

Raskin, A., Boothe, H.H., Reatig, N.A., Schulterbrandt, J.G., and Odle, D. (1971). Factor analyses of normal and depressed patients' memories of parental behavior. *Psychological Reports*, **29,** 871–9.

Reeve, W., and Ivison, D. (1985). Use of environmental manipulation and classroom and modified informal reality orientation with institutionalized, confused elderly patients. *Age and Ageing*, **14,** 119–21.

Regier, D.A., and Burke, J.D. (1988). Population surveys: their relevance to mental health care. In *Handbook of Social Psychiatry* (ed. A.S. Henderson and G.D. Burrows). Elsevier, Amsterdam.

Robins, L.N., Clayton, P.J., and Wing, J.K. (eds) (1980). *The social consequences of psychiatric illness.* Brunner Mazel, New York.

Robins, L.N., Helzer, J.E., Croughan, J., and Ratcliff, K.S. (1981). National

Institute of Mental Health Diagnostic Interview Schedule. Its history, characteristics, and validity. *Archives of General Psychiatry*, **38,** 381–8.

Robins, L.N., Helzer, J.E., Weissman, M.M., Orvaschel, H., Gruenberg, E., Burke, J.D., and Regier, D.A. (1984). Lifetime prevalence of specific psychiatric disorders in three sites. *Archives of General Psychiatry*, **41,** 949–58.

Roe, A., and Siegelman, M. (1963). A parent–child questionnaire. *Child Development*, **34,** 355–69.

Romans-Clarkson, S.E., Clarkson, J.E., Dittmer, I.D., Flett, R., Linsell, C., Mullen, P.E., and Mullin, B. (1986). Impact of a handicapped child on mental health of parents. *British Medical Journal*, **293,** 1395–7.

Rorsman, B., Hagnell, O., and Lanke, J. (1985). Mortality and age psychosis in the Lundby study: death risk of senile and multi-infarct dementia. *Neuropsychobiology*, **14,** 13–16.

Rorsman, B., Hagnell, O., and Lanke, J. (1986). Prevalence and incidence of senile and multi-infarct dementia in the Lundby Study: a comparison between the time periods 1947–1957 and 1957–1972. *Neuropsychobiology*, **15,** 122–9.

Roth, M., Huppert, F.A., Tym, E., and Mountjoy, C.Q. (1988). *CAMDEX: The Cambridge Examination for Mental Disorders of the Elderly*. Cambridge University Press.

Roth, M. *et al.* (1986). CAMDEX. A standardised instrument for the diagnosis of mental disorder in the elderly with special reference to the early detection of dementia. *British Journal of Psychiatry*, **149,** 698–709.

Rutter, M. (1966). *Children of sick parents: An environmental and psychiatric study*. Maudsley Monograph, No. 16. Oxford University Press.

Rutter, M. (1972). *Maternal deprivation reassessed.* Penguin, Harmondsworth.

Rutter, M. (1981). The city and the child. *American Journal of Orthopsychiatry*, **5,** 610–25.

Rutter, M. (1988). Changing patterns of psychiatric disorders over adolescence. In *Adolescence* (ed. J. Bancroft and J. Reinisch). Oxford University Press.

Rutter, M., and Brown, G.W. (1966). The reliability and validity of measures of family life and relationships in families containing a psychiatric patient. *Social Psychiatry*, **1,** 38–53.

Rutter, M., and Hersov, L. (1985). *Child and adolescent psychiatry. Modern approaches*, 2nd edn. Blackwell, Oxford.

Rutter, M., and Quinton, D. (1984). Parental psychiatric disorder: effect on children. *Psychological Medicine*, **14,** 853–80.

Rutter, M., and Sandberg, S. (1985). Epidemiology of child psychiatric disorder: methodological issues and some substantive findings. *Child Psychiatry and Human Development*, **15,** 209–33.

Rutter, M., Yule, W., and Graham, P. (1973). Enuresis and behavioural deviance: some epidemiological considerations. In *Bladder control and enuresis clinics in developmental medicine*, Nos 48/49 (ed. I. Kolvin, R. MacKeith, and S.R. Meadow), pp. 137–47. Heinemann, London.

Rutter, M., Cox, A., Tupling, C., Berger, M., and Yule, W. (1975*a*). Attainment and adjustment in two geographical areas. I. The prevalence of psychiatric disorder. *British Journal of Psychiatry*, **126,** 493–509.

Rutter, M., Yule, B., Quinton, D., Rowlands, O., Yule, W., and Berger, M. (1975*b*). Attainment and adjustment in two geographical areas. III. Some factors accounting for area differences. *British Journal of Psychiatry*, **126,** 520–33.

Rutter, M., Graham, P., Chadwick, O.F.D., and Yule, W. (1976). Adolescent turmoil: fact or fiction? *Journal of Child Psychology and Psychiatry*, **17,** 35–56.

Sackett, D., and Holland, W.W. (1975). Controversy in the detection of disease. *Lancet*, **2,** 357–9.

Sainsbury, P. (1955). *Suicide in London*. Maudsley Monograph Series. Chapman and Hall, London.

Sainsbury, P. (1986). Epidemiology of suicide. In *Suicide* (ed. A. Roy), pp. 17–40. Williams and Wilkins, Baltimore.

Sainsbury, P., Jenkins, J.S., Levey, A., and Baert, A. (1978). *Suicide trends in Europe: A study of the decline in suicide in England and Wales and the increase elsewhere*. World Health Organization Regional Office for Europe, Geneva.

Sanson-Fisher, R.W., and Hennrikus, D.J. (1988). Why do primary care physicians often fail to detect psychological disturbance in their patients? In *Handbook of social psychiatry* (ed. A.S. Henderson and G.D. Burrows). Elsevier, Amsterdam.

Sarason, I.G., and Spielberger, C.D. (1979). *Stress and anxiety*, Vol. 6. Hemisphere, New York.

Sarason, I.G., Levine, H.M., Basham, R.B., and Sarason, B.R. (1983). Assessing social support: the Social Support Questionnaire. *Journal of Personality and Social Psychology*, **44,** 127–39.

Sartorius, N. (1977). Priorities for research likely to contribute to better provision of mental health care. *Social Psychiatry*, **12,** 171–84.

Sartorius, N. (1988). Future directions: a global view. In *Handbook of social psychiatry* (ed. A.S. Henderson and G.D. Burrows). Elsevier, Amsterdam.

Sartorius, N., and Harding, T.W. (1983). The World Health Organization Collaborative Study on Strategies for Extending Mental Health Care, I: The genesis of the study. *American Journal of Psychiatry*, **140,** 1470–3.

Sartorius, N. *et al.* (1986). Early manifestations and first-contact incidence of schizophrenia in different cultures. *Psychological Medicine*, **16,** 909–28.

Sartorius, N., Jablensky, A., Ernberg, G., Leff, J., Korten, A., and Gulbinat,

W. (1987). Course of schizophrenia in different countries: some results of a World Health Organization international comparative 5-year follow-up study. In *Search for the causes of schizophrenia* (ed. H. Hafner, W.F. Gattaz, and W. Janzarik), pp. 107–13. Springer-Verlag, Berlin.

Schaefer, E.S. (1965). A configurational analysis of children's reports of parent behavior. *Journal of Consulting Psychology*, **29,** 552–7.

Scheper-Hughes, N. (1979). *Saints, scholars, and schizophrenics: Mental illness in rural Ireland.* University of California Press, Berkeley.

Schlesselman, J.L. (1982). *Case-control studies: Design, conduct, analysis.* Oxford University Press, New York.

Schoenberg, B.S., Anderson, D.W., and Haerer, A.F. (1981). Prevalence and clinical features of dementia in a biracial population: neuroepidemiological study of a county in rural Mississippi. *Transactions of the American Neurological Association*, **106,** 22–5.

Schradle, S.B., and Dougher, M.J. (1985). Social support as a mediator of stress: theoretical and empirical issues. *Clinical Psychology Review*, **5,** 641–61.

Seligman, M.E.P. (1981). A learned helplessness point of view. In *Behavior therapy for depression: Present status and future directions* (ed. L.P. Rehm), pp. 123–41. Academic Press, New York.

Shepherd, M. (1983). *The psychosocial matrix of psychiatry, collected papers.* Tavistock, London.

Shepherd, M. (1987). Mental illness and primary care. *American Journal of Public Health*, **77,** 12–13.

Shepherd, M., Cooper, B., Brown, A.C., and Kalton, G.W. (1966). *Psychiatric illness in general practice*. Oxford University Press.

Shepherd, M., Cooper, B., Brown, A.C., and Kalton, G.W. (1981). *Psychiatric illness in general practice*. 2nd edn. Oxford University Press.

Shepherd, M., Wilkinson, G., and Williams, P. (1986). *Mental illness in primary care settings*. Tavistock, London.

Shrout, P.E. (1981). Scaling of stressful life events. In *Stressful life events and their contexts* (ed. B.S. Dohrenwend and B.P. Dohrenwend), pp. 29–47. Prodist, New York.

Silberfeld, M. (1978). Psychological symptoms and social supports. *Social Psychiatry*, **13,** 11–17.

Sills, D.L. (ed.) (1968). *International encyclopedia of the social sciences.* Macmillan and The Free Press, New York.

Slater, E. (1943). The neurotic constitution: a statistical study of two thousand soldiers. *Journal of Neurology and Psychiatry*, **6,** 1–16.

Slater, E., and Slater, P. (1944). A heuristic theory of neurosis. *Journal of Neurology and Psychiatry*, **7,** 49–55.

Spector, J. (1984). Clinical psychology and primary care. *Bulletin of the British Psychological Society*, **37,** 73–6.

Srole, L., Langner, T.S., Michael, S.T., Opler, M.K., and Rennie, T.A.C. (1962). *Mental health in the metropolis*, Vol. 1: *The mid-town Manhattan study*. McGraw Hill, New York.

Steele, G.P., Henderson, S., and Duncan-Jones, P. (1980). The reliability of reporting adverse experiences. *Psychological Medicine*, **10,** 301–6.

Stein, Z., and Susser, M. (1969). Widowhood and mental illness. *British Journal of Preventive and Social Medicine*, **23,** 106–10.

Sternberg, E., and Gavrilova, S. (1978). Über klinisch-epidemiologische Untersuchungen in der sowjetischen Alterspsychiatrie. *Nervenarzt*, **49,** 347–53.

Strömgren, E. (1938). Beiträge zur psychischen Erblehre. *Acta Psychiatrica Neurologica*, Supplement 19.

Sturgeon, D., Kuipers, L., Berkowitz, R., Turpin, G., and Leff, J. (1981). Psychophysiological responses of schizophrenic patients to high and low expressed emotion relatives. *British Journal of Psychiatry*, **138,** 40–5.

Sturgeon, D., Turpin, G., Kuipers, L., Berkowitz, R., and Leff, J. (1984). Psychophysiological responses of schizophrenic patients to high and low expressed emotion relatives: a follow-up study. *British Journal of Psychiatry*, **145,** 62–9.

Sulkava, R., Wikstrom, J., Aromaa, A., Raitasalo, R., Lehtinen, V., Lahtela, K., and Palo, J. (1985). Prevalence of severe dementia in Finland. *Neurology*, **35,** 1025–9.

Summers, W.K., Majovski, L.V., Marsh, G.M., Tachiki, K., and Kling, A. (1986). Oral tetrahydroaminoacridine in long-term treatment of senile dementia, Alzheimer type. *New England Journal of Medicine*, **315,** 1242–5.

Surtees, P. (1984). Kith, kin and psychiatric health: a Scottish survey. *Social Psychiatry*, **19,** 63–7.

Surtees, P.G. (1988). Adversity and psychiatric disorder: a decay model. In *Life events and illness: Studies of psychiatric and physical disorders* (ed. G.W. Brown and T. Harris). Guilford Press, New York.

Surtees, P., and Ingham, J. (1980). Life stress and depressive outcome: an application of a dissipation model to life events. *Social Psychiatry*, **15,** 21–31.

Surtees, P.G., Sashidharan, S.P., and Dean C. (1986). Affective disorder amongst women in the general population: a longitudinal study. *British Journal of Psychiatry*, **148,** 176–86.

Susser, M.W., Stein, Z., Mountney, G.H., and Freeman, H.L. (1970*a*). Chronic disability following mental illness in an English city. Part I. Total prevalence in and out of mental hospital. *Social Psychiatry*, **5,** 63–9.

Susser, M.W., Stein, Z., Mountney, G.H., and Freeman, H.L. (1970*b*). Chronic disability following mental illness in an English city. Part II. The location of patients in hospital and community. *Social Psychiatry*, **5,** 69–76.

Tansella, M., de Salvia, D., and Williams, P. (1987). The Italian psychiatric reform: some quantitative evidence. *Social Psychiatry*, **22,** 37–48.

Tansella, M., and Williams, P. (1987). The Italian experience and its implications. *Psychological Medicine*, **17,** 283–9.

Tansella, M., Williams, P., Balestrieri, M., Bellantuono, C., and Martini, N. (1986). The management of affective disorders in the community. *Journal of Affective Disorders*, **11,** 73–9.

Tarrier, N., Vaughn, C., Lader, M.H., and Leff, J.P. (1979). Bodily reactions to people and events in schizophrenia. *Archives of General Psychiatry*, **36,** 311–15.

Taylor, L., and Chave, S. (1964). *Mental health and environment*. Longmans, London.

Tennant, C. (1983). Life events and psychological morbidity: the evidence from prospective studies. *Psychological Medicine*, **13,** 483–6.

Tennant, C.C., (1985*a*). Female vulnerability to depression. *Psychological Medicine*, **15,** 733–7.

Tennant, C.C. (1985*b*). Stress and schizophrenia: a review. *Integrative Psychiatry*, **3,** 248–61.

Tennant, C., and Andrews, G. (1976). A scale to measure the stress of life events. *Australian and New Zealand Journal of Psychiatry*, **10,** 27–32.

Tennant, C., and Andrews, G. (1978). The cause of life events in neurosis. *Journal of Psychosomatic Research*, **22,** 41–5.

Tennant, C., and Bebbington, P. (1978). The social causations of depression: a critique of the work of Brown and his colleagues. *Psychological Medicine*, **8,** 565–75.

Tennant, C., Bebbington, P., and Hurry, J. (1980). Parental death in childhood and risk of adult depressive disorders: a review. *Psychological Medicine*, **10,** 289–299.

Tennant, C., Smith, A., Bebbington, P., and Hurry, J. (1981). Parental loss in childhood: Relationship to adult psychiatric impairment and contact with psychiatric services. *Archives of General Psychiatry*, **38,** 309–14.

Tennant, C., Goulston, G., and Dent, O. (1986*a*). The psychological effects of being a prisoner of war 40 years after release. *American Journal of Psychiatry*, **143,** 618–21.

Tennant, C., Goulston, G., and Dent, O. (1986*b*). Australian prisoners of war of the Japanese—post-war psychiatric hospitalization and psychological morbidity. *Australian and New Zealand Journal of Psychiatry*, **20,** 334–40.

Tennant, C., Goulston, G., and Dent, O. (1986*c*). Clinical psychiatric illness in POWs of the Japanese 40 years after release. *Psychological Medicine*, **16,** 833–9.

Toffler, A. (1971). *Future shock*. Pan, London.

Toffler, A. (1980). *The third wave*. Morrow, New York.

Torrey, E.F. (1980). *Schizophrenia and civilization*, Ch. 2. Aronson, New York.

Turner, R.J., and Wagenfeld, M.O. (1967). Occupational mobility and schizophrenia. *American Sociological Review*, **32,** 104–13.

Vaughn, C.E. (1986). Patterns of emotional response in the families of schizophrenic patients. In *Treatment of schizophrenia: Family assessment and intervention* (ed. M.J. Goldstein, I. Hand, and K. Hahlweg), pp. 97–106. Springer-Verlag, Berlin.

Vaughn, C.E., and Leff, J.P. (1976). The influence of family and social factors on the course of psychiatric illness. *British Journal of Psychiatry*, **129,** 125–37.

Vaughn, C.E., and Leff, J.P. (1981). Patterns of emotional response in relatives of schizophrenic patients. *Schizophrenia Bulletin*, **7,** 43–4.

Vaughn, C.E., Snyder, K., Freeman, W., Jones, S., Falloon, I., and Liberman, R. (1982). Family factors in schizophrenic relapse: a replication. *Schizophrenia Bulletin*, **8,** 425–6.

Vaughn, C.E., Snyder, K.S., Jones, S., Freeman, W.B., and Falloon, I.R.H. (1984). Family factors in schizophrenic relapse. *Archives of General Psychiatry*, **41,** 1169–77.

Vazquez Barquero, J.L., Munoz, P.E., and Madoz Jauregui, V. (1982). The influence of the process of urbanization on the prevalence of neurosis: a community survey. *Acta Psychiatrica Scandinavica*, **65,** 161–70.

Walsh, B., and Grant, M. (1985). *Public health implications of alcohol production and trade*. Offset Publication No. 88. World Health Organization, Geneva.

Walsh, D., and Walsh, B. (1970). Mental illness in the Republic of Ireland: first admissions. *Journal of the Irish Medical Association*, **63,** 365–70.

Walsh, D., O'Hare, A., Blake, B., Halpenny, J.V., and O'Brien, P.F. (1980). The treated prevalence of mental illness in the Republic of Ireland: the Three County Register Study. *Psychological Medicine*, **10,** 465–70.

Warr, P., and Jackson, P. (1985). Factors influencing the psychological impact of prolonged unemployment and of re-employment. *Psychological Medicine*, **15,** 795–807.

Weiss, R.S. (1974). The provisions of social relationships. In *Doing unto others* (ed. Z. Rubin), pp. 17–26. Prentice-Hall, Englewood Cliffs, New Jersey.

Weiss, R.S. (1979). *Going it alone*. Basic Books, New York.

Weiss, R.S. (1982). Attachment in adult life. In *The place of attachment in human behavior* (ed. C.M. Parkes and J. Stevenson-Hinde), pp. 171–84. Basic Books, New York.

Weissman, M.M., and Klerman, G.L. (1977). Sex differences and the epidemiology of depression. *Archives of General Psychiatry*, **34,** 98–111.

Weissman, M.M., Leaf, P.J., Holzer, C.E., Myers, K.J., and Tischler, G.L.

(1984). The epidemiology of depression: an update on sex differences in rates. *Journal of Affective Disorders*, **7**, 179–88.

Weissman, M.M., Myers, J.K., Tischler, G.L., Holzer, C.E., Leaf, P.J., Orvaschel, H., and Brody, J.A. (1985). Psychiatric disorders (DSM–III) and cognitive impairment in the elderly in a U.S. urban community. *Acta Psychiatrica Scandinavica*, **71**, 366–79.

Wells, Y., and Jorm, A.F. (1987). Evaluation of a special nursing home unit for dementia sufferers: *a* randomized controlled comparison with community care. *Australian and New Zealand Journal of Psychiatry*, **21**, 524–31.

Whitehead, A. (1984). Psychological intervention in dementia. In *Handbook of studies on psychiatry and old age* (ed. D.W.K. Kay and G.D. Burrows), pp. 181–99. Elsevier: Amsterdam.

Wig, N.N. *et al.* (1987*a*). Expressed emotion and schizophrenia in North India. I. Cross-cultural transfer of ratings of relatives' expressed emotion. *British Journal of Psychiatry*, **151**, 156–60.

Wig, N.N. *et al.* (1987*b*). Expressed emotion and schizophrenia in North India. II. Distribution of expressed emotion components among relatives of schizophrenic patients in Aarhus and Chandigarh. *British Journal of Psychiatry*, **151**, 160–5.

Wilkin, D. (1979). *Caring for the mentally handicapped child*. Croom Helm, London.

Williams, P. (1986). Mental illness and primary care: screening. In *Mental illness in primary care settings* (ed. M. Shepherd, G. Wilkinson, and P. Williams). Tavistock, London.

Williams, P., Tarnopolsky, A., Hand, D., and Shepherd, M. (1986*a*). Minor psychiatric morbidity and general practice consultations: the West London Survey. *Psychological Medicine*, Monograph Supplement No. 9.

Williams, P., de Salvia, D., and Tansella, M. (1986*b*). Suicide, psychiatric reform, and the provision of psychiatric services in Italy. *Social Psychiatry*, **21**, 89–95.

Williamson, J. *et al.* (1964). Old people at home: their unreported needs. *Lancet*, **1**, 1117–20.

Wing, J.K. (1966). Social and psychological changes in a rehabilitation unit. *Social Psychiatry*, **1**, 21–8.

Wing, J.K. (1972). Principles of evaluation. In *Evaluating a community psychiatric service: The Camberwell Register, 1964–1971* (ed. J.K. Wing and A.M. Hailey), pp. 11–39. Oxford University Press.

Wing, J.K. (1973). The social context of schizophrenia. *American Journal of Psychiatry*, **135**, 1333–9.

Wing, J.K. (ed.) (1975). *Schizophrenia from within*. National Schizophrenia Fellowship, London.

Wing, J.K. (ed.) (1978*a*). *Schizophrenia: Towards a new synthesis*. Academic Press, London.

Wing, J.K. (1978*b*). *Reasoning about madness*. Oxford University Press.

Wing, J.K. (ed.) (1982). Long-term community care: experience in a London borough. *Psychological Medicine*, **12,** Supplement 2, 1–97.

Wing, J.K., and Brown, G.W. (1961). Social treatment of chronic schizophrenia: a comparative survey of three mental hospitals. *Journal of Mental Science*, **107,** 847–61.

Wing, J.K., and Brown, G.W. (1970). *Institutionalism and schizophrenia*. Cambridge University Press.

Wing, J.K., and Freudenberg, R.K. (1961). The response of severely ill chronic schizophrenic patients to social stimulation. *American Journal of Psychiatry*, **118,** 311–22.

Wing, J.K., and Hafner, H. (eds) (1973). *Roots of evaluation. The epidemiological basis for planning psychiatric services*. Oxford University Press.

Wing, J.K., and Hailey, A.M. (eds.) (1972). *Evaluating a community psychiatric service*. Oxford University Press.

Wing, J.K., Monck, E., Brown, G.W., and Carstairs, G.M. (1964). Morbidity in the community of schizophrenic patients discharged from London mental hospitals in 1959. *British Journal of Psychiatry*, **110,** 10–21.

Wing, J.K., Cooper, J.E., and Sartorius, N. (1974). *The description of psychiatric symptoms: An introduction manual for the PSE and CATEGO system*. Cambridge University Press.

Wing, J.K., Nixon, J., Von Cranach, M., and Strauss, A. (1977). Further developments of the 'Present State Examination' and CATEGO System. *Archives of Psychiatry and Neurological Sciences*, **22,** 151–60.

Wing, J.K., Bebbington, P., and Robins, L.N. (1981). *What is a case? The problem of definitions in psychiatric community surveys*. Grant McIntyre, London.

Wolman, B.J. (ed.) (1973). *Dictionary of behavioural science*. Macmillan, London.

Woods, R.T. (1979). Reality orientation and staff attention: a controlled study. *British Journal of Psychiatry*, **134,** 502–7.

World Health Organization (1968). *Prevention of suicide*. Public Health Paper No. 35. World Health Organization, Geneva.

World Health Organization (1977). *Forensic psychiatry. Report of a working group*. Regional Office for Europe, World Health Organization, Copenhagen.

World Health Organization (1979). *Schizophrenia. An international follow-up study*. World Health Organization; Wiley, Chichester.

World Health Organization (1980). *International classification of impairments, disabilities, and handicaps. A manual of classification relating to the consequences of disease*. World Health Organization, Geneva.

World Health Organization (1982*a*). *Changing patterns in suicide behaviour*.

Report on a World Health Organization working group. Euro Reports and Studies no. 74. World Health Organization, Copenhagen.

World Health Organization (1982*b*). *Epidemiological studies on social and medical conditions of the elderly*. Euro Report Series, 62, Regional Office for Europe, Copenhagen.

World Health Organization (1984). *The uses of epidemiology in the study of the elderly*. Report of a World Health Organization Scientific Group on the Epidemiology of Aging, Technical Report Series 706. World Health Organization, Geneva.

World Health Organization (1985*a*). *Dementia in later life: Research and action*. Report of a World Health Organization Scientific Group on Senile Dementia. Technical Report Series, No. 730. World Health Organization, Geneva.

World Health Organization (1985*b*). *Prevention of mental, neurological and psychosocial disorders*. Report by the Director-General, World Health Organization to the 77th session of the Executive Board.

Yap, P.M. (1974). *Comparative psychiatry: A theoretical framework* (ed. M.P. Lau and A.B. Stokes). University of Toronto Press.

Young, M., Bernard, B., and Wallis, G. (1963). The mortality of widowers. *Lancet*, **2,** 454–6.

Zimmermann-Tansella, C., Burti, L., Faccincani, C., Garzotto, N., Siciliani, O., and Tansella, M. (1985). Bringing into action the psychiatric reform in South-Verona. A five year experience. *Acta Psychiatrica Scandinavica*, 71 Supplement, **316,** 71–86.

Zung, W.W.K. (1965). A self-rating depression scale. *Archives of General Psychiatry*, **12,** 63–70.

Author index

Subject Index